Praise for
HOPE FIGHTS BACK

"Despite the limitations imposed by ALS, Andrea shatters the belief that it hampers her achievements and being. She gives hope to so many that have lost it. *Hope Fights Back* is full of optimism, positivity, and strength. Its profound message serves as a powerful reminder for all of us to seize every waking moment and make the most of our lives."

—Mike Reilly, the Voice of IRONMAN,
USA Triathlon Hall of Fame

"Although her time is limited by ALS, Andrea lives her life without limits. When so many would lose hope, instead Andrea's fighting spirit burns like a fire. One cannot read her jaw-dropping story without feeling utterly inspired, determined to seize every opportunity and make the most of every moment we have."

—Chrissie Wellington, OBE,
four-time IRONMAN World Champion

"Andrea Peet is an example of what happens when hope is met with passion and perseverance. Her story is an inspiration to all of us."

—Tony Hawk, Professional Skateboarder

"What is the purpose of hope? Andrea Lytle Peet shines a light on this question as she details accepting life with ALS. In her story, at times heartbreaking and humorous, we can all find lessons on how to move forward with intention, even against the current. *Hope Fights Back* inspires and celebrates the beauty of choice."

—Sarah Gearhart, author of *We Share the Sun*

HOPE FIGHTS BACK

HOPE FIGHTS BACK

FIFTY MARATHONS AND A LIFE-OR-DEATH RACE AGAINST ALS

ANDREA LYTLE PEET
WITH MEREDITH ATWOOD

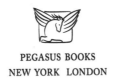

PEGASUS BOOKS
NEW YORK LONDON

HOPE FIGHTS BACK

Pegasus Books, Ltd.
148 West 37th Street, 13th Floor
New York, NY 10018

Copyright © 2023 by Andrea Lytle Peet and Meredith Atwood

First Pegasus Books cloth edition September 2023

Interior design by Maria Fernandez

Interior swallow illustrations by James Atwood IV

Library of Congress Cataloging-in-Publication Data is available.

ISBN: 978-1-63936-477-0

10 9 8 7 6 5 4 3 2 1

Printed in the United States of America
Distributed by Simon & Schuster
www.pegasusbooks.com

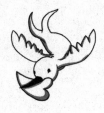

For David

My person

CONTENTS

PART III: HOPE FIGHTS BACK

INTRODUCTION

ALS

The simplest things in life are not simple for everyone.

An average, healthy person doesn't think about getting up from a chair to pour themselves a glass of water.

Instead, that person might think, *I'm thirsty*. But the next part? Well, it's quite automatic.

The person uses their legs to push the chair back. They stand up, walk over to the cabinet in the kitchen, reach for a glass, and fill it with the tap. Or maybe they like their water bottled or sparkling in a can. So instead of reaching for a glass, they twist off a cap, pop a lid.

Ultimately, they lift the glass or bottle or can to their mouth. They take a swig, maybe say "ahhhhh!" like on a cheesy commercial, and return to their seat.

Or they might carry the water back to their seat—where they place it on the table, sit down, and resume doing whatever thing they were doing before the semiconscious thought *I'm thirsty*.

All these actions occurred before the person thought too much about anything. And it took maybe thirty seconds to accomplish.

The process is easy. They're no longer thirsty and have since moved on to the next task at hand. The same thing can be said about brushing teeth, eating, and even driving.

But for someone with ALS, the simplest things are no longer taken for granted—because they are no longer simple. A body with ALS has long refused to respond automatically—to most anything. Each movement is labored, well thought out, and debated as to whether it's even worth the effort to *try*. And then, some movements are impossible—or will be impossible in a matter of time.

Someone with ALS must tell their body every single action to take to get from the chair to the kitchen to carefully swallowing the water. It probably eats up five frustrating minutes of the life they know is speeding toward its end.

That is—if they're still lucky enough to be walking, drinking water, or even breathing on their own . . .

So, let's break it down.

To move *any* muscle in your body, two nerve connections must occur.

When the average person thinks *I'm thirsty*, the body begins to send messages internally—just from the thought itself.

This messaging is so rapid that the process of getting up and grabbing some water is instantaneous and almost unconscious. In other words, you had the thought to quench the thirst, so you're now simply *doing it*.

In a healthy body, the brain quickly sends a message to the spinal cord through what are called the *upper* motor neurons. Then, the *lower* motor neurons respond to this message. This is how the getting-up-and-walking happens—when both the upper and lower neurons "talk" to each other.

This upper-lower neuron messaging repeats all day long when doing most everything in a healthy body: a rapid-fire process of brushing your teeth, lifting your arms, reaching into a cabinet, filling the glass—and so on.

Amyotrophic lateral sclerosis,[1] commonly known as ALS or Lou Gehrig's disease, basically causes the upper and lower motor neurons to stop talking to each other.

The effect on the lower motor neurons is what makes ALS deadly. The body's muscles no longer receive the signals to move, so the muscles simply stop moving.

Eventually, the muscles atrophy from lack of use.

Because the lungs are muscles, most people with ALS die of respiratory failure within two to five years of diagnosis.

But not everyone . . .

⟨≈⟩

My name is Andrea Peet. I am forty-two years old, and I have been living with ALS for nine years.

Before my ALS diagnosis, I had become an adult-onset athlete. I loved to swim and bike and run, and the challenges the sports presented when combined into a triathlon. At the time, I worried mostly about my running pace and how my triathlon suit fit.

I had no idea what was to come—mentally, physically, and beyond.

After my diagnosis, I went through the stages of everything. There are many, many stages—not a set number of them—when one is faced with dying.

Hope is easily and unknowingly abandoned in times of fear and illness, loss and grief. The immediate goal becomes Acceptance—as in, accepting that whatever future is to come must be written in the stars, happening for a reason.

I went through basic Acceptance. I accepted that I would die—a fact that everyone will face eventually, whether we like to think about it or not.

But then, with Acceptance came the desire to do one last race before my body failed me. So, I finished one more triathlon—and well, crossing that finish line changed everything. I am beyond lucky.

Acceptance took on a new meaning. I could accept I had ALS. I also accepted that my journey through the disease could inspire others, and therefore leave a lasting impact on the world. With that, a feeling of Hope crept in and began to drive the journey to some unexpected destinations.

Oddly, I discovered I could still accomplish physical goals—even with the death sentence of ALS hanging over me. My legs—although quite rebellious when it came to walking—were pretty fan-freaking-tastic at pedaling an adorable three-wheeled bike—better known as a trike. More on that later.

Out of this *ability* to pedal came the birth of a dream.

I would not wait around for this disease to kill me.

I could not "run," but I *could* still race.

I could still live.

So, on my trike, I set a goal to finish fifty marathons in fifty states, pedaling with my own power. The beginning of that dream started in 2015 and took off in 2019 as we launched a documentary film project. I was well on my way until the COVID-19 pandemic shut down the world. I wasn't sure how I could make those remaining marathons happen in *all* the states when everything, including marathons, was canceled.

Time was limited, and I knew my time, especially, had limits.

As I said before, most people with ALS live two to five years after diagnosis. When the pandemic started, I had already lived six years with ALS. Could I really expect to live long enough—and maintain the strength needed—to complete the remaining thirty-three marathons?

Spoiler alert: I finished that fiftieth marathon on May 28, 2022—the start of my eighth year with ALS. Actually, I finished fifty-one marathons. More on that later, too.

I fought for every mile and milestone, every single day since my weird, confusing diagnosis process began. I fought to learn how to live in the face of death. I learned to love, to communicate, and to cherish the relationships in my life in new ways.

I learned to let go of guilt. This is a big one for me.

This book is the only way I can still tell my story as thoroughly as I'd like. My voice can only handle a few breathy sentences at a time these days, so I am grateful you are here to read all the words I need to write to share my story.

In this journey, I have learned that Hope is not a delicate, sweet thing. Rather, Hope is powerful. Hope isn't weak. Hope isn't timid.

Hope is a badass and brave warrior.

My story is one of sadness, fear, laughter, and love.

But really, it is a story about what happens when Hope Fights Back.

With love,
Andrea

P.S.
Go on, be brave. End ALS.

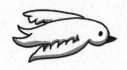

PART I

HOPE
IS
LOST

CHAPTER 1
THE STUCK FINGER

Pre-diagnosis: January 2013

The foreshadowing of my death appeared in my right index finger.

It was a freezing January morning in Washington, DC, and I was swimming in a brightly lit indoor pool. To motivate myself, I pretended I was in a sparkling ocean somewhere exotic with the sun shining down. It helped.

My father-in-law, Dr. Dave, and I were swim training for our next triathlon. (Dr. Dave is not to be confused with my husband—*David*—who is a lawyer, not a doctor.)

My entire body glided through the silky warm water—but not my right index finger. I swam smoothly with grace. Except for that finger staging a vicious, strange, and ridiculous protest.

Come on, finger, get with the program.

I imagined an "off" day for an index finger was a rare thing—probably even rarer to notice such a minute detail. But it was distracting and throwing off my swim game.

I reached over the swim rope during a lap break and showed Dr. Dave.

"It's weird," I said, pulling my goggles onto my forehead. "I can't fully extend my finger when I take a stroke. It's, like, stuck or something."

He pulled off his goggles and squinted. My hand looked like a crooked old-lady hand—all pruned up from the swim *and* with that odd, stubbornly bent finger.

Dr. Dave wiggled my fingers a few times. He shook the water out of his ears.

"Huh. Well, we could tape your fingers together?" Family doctors and fathers-in-law are clearly not prone to alarm.

"Nah," I said.

I returned my goggles to my face. I decided to finish the swim strong. Which I did. But the finger didn't quite get unstuck until hours later.

Looking back, it was the first sign of ALS. The very first breadcrumb in a long, miserable trail of questions leading to the definitive answer: *You are going to die.*

I was thirty-one years old that day and had no idea that a "stuck" finger was the beginning of the end. The beginning of a life changed abruptly and forever. The beginning of my search for meaning and purpose.

⟨⟩

It seems narcissistic or idiotic now, but honestly, I had never given death any thought.

I didn't believe I was invincible. I simply believed I had time. That there would always be enough time, enough hours, enough hugs and kisses, more triathlons and countless marathons to look forward to.

I lived with the expectation of a classically beautiful, long life with my husband, David. There would be kids—who knew how many or when—but kids were in the expectation, the vision. And after we retired, maybe I'd learn to knit or start playing the French horn again. Maybe I would do 5Ks with the grandkids. They'd exclaim, "Wow, Grandma. You are fast!"

Or maybe I'd be crotchety and point with my little-old-lady finger while saying "Get off my lawn!"

A bent finger in the pool. A crooked old-lady finger. The start of my perfect little-old-lady dream life disintegrating before my eyes.

CHAPTER 2

THE CHECKLIST

Childhood: Sometime in 1991

When I was ten years old, I read about myself in a magazine.

At the pediatrician's office, Mom decided I was old enough to see the doctor alone—just in case I wanted to discuss any pre-puberty questions with her. *I did not want to do any such thing. Gross.*

I didn't have any period questions, but I did feel a teensy bit more grown-up as I followed the nurse to the exam room. As soon as the door closed, I scurried out of my clothes and into the crinkly paper gown before anyone could catch me in my underwear.

Safely seated in my paper gown, I scanned my reading options. *Ugh.* All the books were for little kids. So, I settled for a parenting magazine.

Flipping through, a checklist caught my attention. The headline read something like: Real Traits of Only Children. *Hey, that's me!*

I perused the list:

1. Mature beyond their age? *Check.*
2. Eager to please? *Yes, ma'am.*

3. Acts like a little adult? *Well, now that you mention it . . .*
4. Confident? *Yep.*
5. Plays well by themself? *Uh-huh.*
6. Does well in school? *Duh.*
7. Hard on themself? *Oh, good god, yes.*

I sat back, slightly appalled. How did a magazine know that much about me—just because I had no siblings?

But the checklist *was* me—my personality distilled into list form. All this time, I believed I was special and unique, just like my parents told me.

But something clicked the day I found the magazine. The checklist "about me" gave me the framework to explain myself *to* myself throughout the confusion of middle and high school.

Why did I invite friends over to write a letter to our middle school band director about the discipline problems in class? *Because I'm an only child and therefore mature for my age and act like a little adult.*

Why was I such a goody-goody who never smoked, drank, or cut class? *Because I'm an only child and eager to please.*

Why was I taking five Advanced Placement classes even though I was completely lost in the material, totally stressed out, and unlikely to score high enough on the test to earn college credit? *Because I'm an only child and supposed to do well in school. And let's not forget, hard on myself.*

In AP English, I read Nietzsche's quote "What does not kill you makes you stronger."[1] I adopted it as my personal mantra and badge of honor. I would have tattooed it on my face, but goody-goodies don't get tattoos.

What does not kill you makes you stronger.

Apparently, both Nietzsche and I were wrong.

I have since learned that what kills you will make you simultaneously weaker and stronger, more alive yet closer to dead, beating up your mobility but ever-increasing your ability, shrinking your muscles and growing your heart, killing your plans but expanding your dreams.

Crap. That's entirely too much to tattoo on my face.

Above all, the parenting magazine checklist explained why I'd always pictured myself as a little-kid version of my parents. And why not? They were good, hardworking people who loved me—and each other—endlessly. We were a unit, a package deal.

Discovering we were actually three separate people, each with our own flaws, blind spots, and unique journeys? Well, *that* realization led to all sorts of conflict, guilt, and heartache.

⊂⊃

Mom and Dad were married eighteen years before I was born.

They got married three days after Mom's eighteenth birthday in 1963. "After choir practice," as Mom tells the story. "Your dad stayed up all night trying to talk me into marrying him." I thought that was so romantic.

Mom (real name: Sandy) hadn't even finished high school at the time. She started dating Dad (real name: Andy) after squirting him with a hose at a church car wash.

Sandy was a freshman; Andy was a senior. She was a Girl Scout; he was a Boy Scout. Sandy's dad had died the year before; Andy made her laugh again.

That's right, Sandy and Andy—a pair of rhyming romantics.

While Sandy was in high school, Andy joined the Coast Guard, leading to a long-distance courtship for four years.

In April 1963, Sandy visited Andy in Maine over Easter break—along with his parents, of course. Andy laid out the "marry me" argument logically: his enlistment was almost up, and she had almost graduated high school. They were in love. Everything else could be figured out.

The very next day, a Thursday, Andy's minister married them in a room inside the Presbyterian church. His parents and youngest brother were there, along with the choir, and their good friends, Mary and Jerry (I am not kidding).

Sandy wore the peach-colored knit suit she had brought for an Easter dress. Afterward, they called Sandy's mom.

("Do not do this," Mom always says at this point in her retelling of the story.)

My grandmother, Anna, was more relieved than anything. Anna had lived through the Depression and survived on her skills of sewing, gardening, and canning for winter. But as resourceful as she was, it was hard to make ends meet after her husband died. Sandy was the youngest of five children and twenty years younger than her eldest sibling—who was already having kids of her own.

No wonder Sandy was ready to get out of Ohio.

"I saw the writing on the wall," she always told me. "The women in my family got pregnant and they never got to go to college. And that's why I got on birth control."

"Mom!" I'd say, rolling my eyes.

They moved to a little summer cottage outside Freeport, Maine. A cute house and beautiful setting on a tidal river. But once winter hit, they learned why it was affordable. The temperature *in the house* dipped so far below zero that the water in the toilet bowl froze. Dad had to ram his fist through the ice to get it to flush. Twice.

The final straw (icicle?) broke when Mom started up the VW Beetle and the gear shift snapped off in her hand. That's how brittle the metal had become in sub-thirty-degree weather. The prospect of freezing to death wasn't enough to move them, but the cost of car repair was.

They moved back to an apartment in Freeport proper. Even still, throughout their remaining winters in Maine, Dad removed the car battery and brought it inside each night to avoid any more costly car repairs.

"The winters in Maine were why we went to Australia," Dad says.

(Australia stories are my favorite Andy and Sandy stories.)

In 1968, Dad brought home a *Life* magazine and flipped it open to an advertisement with a man wearing a cap and gown walking along the beach. The ad said that the Australian government wanted young American professionals to move to Australia to help with their ongoing shortage of teachers and tradespeople.

At the time, Dad was finishing college with a degree in industrial arts and plans to teach. Mom was a dental assistant. The dentist she worked for was a terrible man who routinely made his staff—and occasionally patients—cry. Mom held the record for grit and longevity. She needed the job, so she learned to anticipate which tools to hand him at which precise moment, and to ignore his moods. This last skill would come in handy later in life with her daughter.

It was a gamble to use their small savings and begin a new life on the other side of the world, but they were determined. They had learned to trust their ability to work hard.

"This is why we don't have a bunch of salt in our food," Mom often says at the dinner table. "We couldn't afford it then, so we don't need it now."

Once they found jobs, their four years in Sydney were relatively simple. Mom worked for a prosthodontist, and Dad was a teacher at an all-boys high school perched on the cliffs near the entrance to Sydney Harbor. After each workday ended, Dad rode his bike down the hill toward Bondi Beach with a surfboard under his arm. Surfing and swimming were free. Mom sewed matching orange-and-brown swimsuits for them. Dad already knew how to fix everything on their new (used) VW Beetle, but it didn't break down nearly as much without the harsh Maine winters.

I might have been born an Aussie if not for my grandmother's lung cancer. Upon her diagnosis, my parents prepared to return to Ohio to take care of her. But before they left, word came that she had passed away. Rather than killing her slowly, her cigarettes went with a more direct route: a fire. She died smoking in bed.

"And this is why you should never smoke. Well, one of the reasons," Mom says.

Horrified and sad, but practical always, Andy and Sandy faced a choice. There was no reason to race back to America, but they had already dismantled their lives in Australia. After much discussion and recalculating of savings, they bought tickets aboard a ship to Cape Town, South Africa. For the next eight months, they traveled across the continent of Africa (a whole other set of Andy and Sandy stories that are too much for this book).

Back in the States, Dad finished his master's degree, and then it was Mom's turn. "I always knew I wanted to go to college before I had a child," she says. "Because the women in my family got pregnant and then they—"

"I *knowwwwww*," I interrupt.

I heard these stories so many times growing up, they became my own personal edition of *Grimms' Fairy Tales*. I knew *alllll* the lessons coming with each tale. I absorbed them long ago.

Hard work is how Andy and Sandy got to live in Australia. Hard work is how they managed to tour around Africa when they started out too poor to afford salt. So yes, I think my personality and work ethic makes a lot of sense after all.

By middle school, I knew I wasn't the smartest kid in class, but I could outwork them all. Because that was the family way.

CHAPTER 3

ADULT-ONSET ATHLETE

Pre-diagnosis: January 2010

Three years before I officially started dying, I started running. Thanks to a *lie*. Or let's call it a *sweeping generalization* that turned out to be flat wrong.

"Don't worry," my new husband, David, said when I moved from Atlanta to Washington, DC, to begin our married life. "It never snows in DC."

We were hit by three blizzards in six weeks. The first blizzard transformed my new city into a brilliant white palace when the sun came out.

During the second blizzard, we made vast quantities of chili and played bad pool in our apartment building's rec room.

By the third blizzard, I was tired of snow, tired of chili, and tired of being cooped up in our little apartment. I needed to *move*. I threw on a T-shirt, shorts, and a pair of sneakers and announced to David that I was going for a run on the treadmill downstairs.

"Do you know where it is?" A fair question.

"I'll find it," I said, and skipped out the door.

Fifteen minutes later, sweating and gasping for air, I hit the button to decrease the speed to a jog, then a walk. Even with my heart pounding and breathing heavy, I felt awake and alive in a way I hadn't felt since I was a kid. *I could do this every single day!*

I had never been an athlete. I had been a coxswain for the crew (rowing) team in college. My job was to steer the boat, lead workout drills, and yell at the four men as they rowed.

Back then, I was so small and thin that we had to carry a sack of sand in the boat during races so our team didn't have an unfair advantage. *One! Two! Three!* I was a tiny, unathletic dictator, shouting orders to the real athletes. *One! Two! Three!* I loved being in charge, but also not in charge whatsoever. *Parenting Magazine Checklist Item Number . . .*

Away from the crushing weight of classes, assignments, fraternities, and all the rest that college demanded, the four men and their petite drill sergeant could focus on one thing only: perfecting the stroke to make the oars click in unison—*thunk*—each and every time. The boat must be level on the water, no one digging an oar deeper in the water than anyone else—a trying task for sleep-deprived college students to pull off at dawn, but a thrill when it happened.

As coxswain, I learned to sense the errors with each stroke, even lying down in the front of the boat facing forward, not looking at the men or their oars. We were a club team without a coach, so I put myself in charge. *Parenting Magazine Checklist Item Number . . .*

Eventually, I could feel which team member was catching late, who was digging, who was rushing the slide. I issued the correction through my headset microphone to the speaker by the stroke seat, all the way down the boat. I tried to balance out the bossy-pantsness with a steady stream of encouragement.

"Great job guys, coming up on five hundred meters to go. You've got this! Starboard side, one of y'all is catching late—I think it's David. Let's take ten strokes to focus on the catch. *Now!* Here we go: *One! Two! Three! . . .*"

Yes, I said David. I spent a whole semester with my future husband in my boat, screaming at him and correcting him over and over, and our relationship not only survived, but appeared to thrive. That's either a great testament to our love—or that he got used to my nagging from the outset.

When things clicked on the boat, I quieted down. Those were the most treasured times on the water—not because *I* was silent, but because *the world* was silent. (Although, if you asked my teammates, perhaps they would say it was because I stopped yelling.) The slick calm of the water as our boat sliced through the stillness. The hollow, rhythmic *thunk* of the oars. The morning rose up and all around us. From my position lying in the bow, just inches from the water, I had a front-row seat to the magic show: the dark sky warming from gray to pink in the predawn, perfectly mirrored in the water.

Except for the oars, all pulling together, the world was truly silent.

When the snow melted in DC, I started running outside. The rhythmic, hypnotic beat of my shoes hitting the pavement in the early morning reminded me of the peace and the oars on the lake. My feet were the oars, my body the boat, and the pavement my own personal lake.

And I was the boss of me.

Exploring the city on foot came in handy for my job as an urban planner. After grad school, I'd snagged the coolest job I never knew existed: working for a federal agency charged with overseeing the government's massive footprint in the nation's capital. Teeming with complex, messy issues and heated politics, it was the perfect learning laboratory for a nerdy do-gooder like me. As a recent transplant to DC, running helped me learn the layout of the city and check out the latest controversial development projects.

Growing up in the suburbs of Raleigh, North Carolina, I assumed everyone drove everywhere—all over the world. Until I went to Davidson College, a small liberal arts school situated in a picturesque little downtown. I was amazed that I could *walk* to the post office, public library, and coffee shop. No need for a car. *Why aren't all cities like this?* I thought. This was before I realized that cities are the by-product of millions of incremental decisions made by actual *people*.

Once I connected those dots, I knew I'd found my career path.

From that point on, cities fascinated me. Streetscapes, parking, transit access, affordable housing, economic development, all of it. What works, what doesn't, and why. And there was no better way to experience a city than during a nice, long run.

I worked up to my first marathon in 2012.

The work ethic from Andy and Sandy fell into place when the idea of a finish line got involved. A goal! Now that made sense to me. Signing up for a race distance just slightly out of reach scared me enough to follow a training plan—and made me feel guilty for missing a workout. Ah, fear and guilt. Such great motivators.

The technique of terrifying myself into disciplined training worked like a charm when I got into triathlons.

I hadn't been swimming regularly since little-kid swim team, so I took swim lessons. The only motivation I needed to improve my swimming ability was picturing a body of water with no pool wall to grab onto. For cycling motivation, I pictured DC's traffic building up at morning rush hour. That image was scary enough to roll me out of bed and get me (and my bike) to the trail—early.

On Christmas morning 2012, I unwrapped a present from David—a package of red T-shirts with TEAM DREA emblazoned in lime-green letters—with silhouettes of a figure swimming, biking, and running. One T-shirt each for me, David, Andy, and Sandy.

I smiled big at David. "Drea" has been his nickname for me since college.

"2013 will be the Year of the Triathlon," he announced, beaming.

I squealed. It was the perfect gift.

My job had been crazy over the past year, and I needed to set some boundaries—a reason to leave the office. Training would be a great way to set new, productive, and healthy limitations. I wanted to sign up for a 70.3-mile triathlon (also known as a half-distance triathlon)—a race consisting of a 1.2-mile swim, 56-mile bike, and 13.1-mile run.

This so-called Year of the Triathlon represented a reset button for me, a chance to redefine myself as a *real* athlete, and to restore a clear work-life balance.

I dove headfirst into triathlon training in January 2013. That's why I was swimming with my father-in-law when I first noticed my stuck finger. My triathlon dream was just a baby when that small foreshadowing of death cast its shadow.

CHAPTER 4

SHAKY LEGS

Pre-diagnosis: September 2013

My half-distance triathlon took place at Davidson College, our alma mater, in North Carolina. Arriving at Davidson's lake campus before dawn reminded me of all those early-morning crew practices. But instead of shouting at David and the other guys, I was the athlete now. It wasn't our boat slicing through the slick, calm water; it was me, swimming. I had used this vision over and over during my swim workouts. It calmed me. Whatever was happening at work or with my stress over the race, the underwater world was silent. Gliding through the water became a meditation, punctuated by a perfect, rhythmic stroke. Only *I* chose when to break that silence to issue a correction or an encouragement to myself. *I was that powerful.*

On race morning, I wrote "Be Brave" on my forearm in Sharpie. I had no idea just how much bravery I would soon need.

The swim started and ended before I knew it. Climbing out of the lake, I took one last glance over my shoulder at the buoys. *Did I really just swim that far?* I paused for a grateful second to absorb my accomplishment before facing the next challenge: the bike. My nemesis.

Unlike swimming, where I could feel my progress week after week, training on the bike had gone in the wrong direction. As the distance on the bike grew, my pace slowed—even with extra indoor cycling classes. And I couldn't make a timely escape from my clipped-in pedals when rolling to a stop—which resulted in many slow-motion tip-overs in DC traffic. To be honest, I had some ugly self-talk going on in my head when I rode my bike.

During the 70.3, there weren't many bikes left in the transition area by the time I mounted mine. *Great, like I wasn't already worried about the cutoff time.* Up and down the hills, I pedaled steadily, finding my rhythm, shifting through the gears. I was encouraged with every passing mile. *I am not fast, but I am doing this!*

Coming into the bike-to-run transition area, my legs shook uncontrollably—I assumed from being on the bike for almost four hours. A race volunteer caught the front of my bike and helped me off. When he noticed my shakes, he walked with me to make sure I was okay.

In reality, the leg shaking had been happening for months. Like in the shower when I propped my foot up on the side of the tub to shave. Or when I raced down the Metro escalator trying to catch a train.

A few other weird things happened that summer. Hints so subtle that I only understood them in retrospect. I found myself exasperated when I spotted a slip of paper on our apartment's mailbox indicating a package for pickup. For some reason, filling out the mail form had become a burden. *Is my handwriting getting slower?*

Or when I worked from home with headphones, the sudden ding in my ear of my cell phone or someone joining a conference call made me jump. My jump would cause the wireless mouse to skitter off the table, causing the cat to jump. This happened several times a day. *Man, I really need to calm down.*

My mind focused back on the race. I needed to stay calm for the run, too.

I passed the miles on the run course checking out the new buildings and businesses—development built since I interned for the Town of Davidson's planning department a decade before. The drawings on paper from back then had come to life.

The course wound onto Davidson College's cross-country trails. Since I hadn't run in college, I had no idea the gravel trails were so hilly.

I was forced to walk every downhill. My hamstrings and calves had been tight for weeks, but completely stiffened as I ran. My sense of balance seemed off too, threatening to pitch me forward onto my face. *It must be all the training. Nine workouts a week is a lot for anyone.*

I was tired of the syrupy sweetness of my energy gels and the Gatorade at the aid stations. I was tired of running. Tired of exercising, tired of moving. Tired of worrying about how slow I was and if I would finish in under eight hours. *Just get there. Then you can rest.*

Eventually, I rounded a corner and saw the inflatable finish line arch. I propelled myself toward it through sheer will. My mind *made* my muscles run.

I finished. All smiles and unbelievably proud of the medal hanging around my neck, but I was a bit embarrassed about being one of the last ones out on the course. *There will be more,* I promised myself. I will get faster. More, faster. I had time.

If I had only known what was coming, I might have slowed down—not with racing, but in the hurried pursuit of all things in my life.

I might have realized that a crooked finger and shaky legs were only the beginning.

And I might have paused at that finish line arch for a moment longer to enjoy my accomplishment.

CHAPTER 5

GUANTANAMO
AND A GOLDFISH

Pre-diagnosis: November 2013

I rested six weeks after my half-distance triathlon, but my problems with balance and shaky legs continued to worsen. Tight hamstrings, too, which showed up in full force at my next running race—eight miles as part of a relay team in Raleigh's City of Oaks Marathon.

Even without all the swimming and biking beforehand, I had to walk every downhill or risk face-planting on the pavement. *This is a really weird injury. I've got to get this checked out.*

I scheduled a screening with a physical therapist, Kerry, an accomplished triathlete.

She took video of me walking on the treadmill. About twenty seconds in, she lowered her phone and stared. I knew why. I was walking like a toddler. My feet too wide apart, my steps uneven.

"I'm going to refer you to a neurologist, just to be safe," she said, her gaze not quite meeting mine. "I'm being conservative, but I want to make sure there's not an underlying problem going on."

I nodded.

Quietly, she added, "Your muscles don't seem strong enough for someone who just did a half-distance triathlon."

Well, shit, I thought on the way home. *Another appointment. More time away from work.*

I became obsessed with watching people walk. Whether in pumps or sneakers or loafers, I noticed toes flex upward slightly just before they stepped down. Everyone's toes—without them thinking about it—did the flex upward thing. *How have I never noticed this before?*

I tried copying them, walking with my toes flexing upward. Yes, I could do it. But I had to concentrate to make it happen. Concentrating to walk? That was certainly new.

But I could do it. I was that type of person. I could do anything if I worked hard enough—even walking correctly.

⚬

Between end-of-the-year deadlines, holiday happy hours, and Christmas shopping, I did not think much about the neurologist appointment scheduled for mid-December.

Anyway, I was far more interested in my ob-gyn appointment the week before the neurologist.

David accompanied me to the ob-gyn. We planned to discuss stopping birth control and conducting genetic testing before trying for a baby. As an only child, I hadn't been around babies much. Still, I assumed kids were in my future—inevitable, like finishing high school or getting a job. *Check.* Just another stepping stone in life, just another monumental privilege I had taken for granted.

Not until I fell in love with David did I truly *want* a child.

He would be a loving and attentive dad. I could tell from the way he played with our niece and nephew. Heck, I could tell from the way he cared for our *cat.* A baby would be a culmination of our love; a precious little human we could pour love into.

When I mentioned the neurology appointment at the end of our ob-gyn visit, the doctor said, "Oh no, I don't think that will interfere with anything. Have fun, kids!"

But a week later, as David and I sat across from the neurologist, I began to get nervous.

Dr. Hampton was pretty, with far more fashion sense than I had. A pretty doctor—okay, fine—but a *fashionable* one? No. A doctor should be pale and nerdy looking, reflecting all their years of serious, devoted study to healing people and putting them back together. Right? Okay, maybe not.

But I needed to focus on something other than how my hands were suddenly shaking.

As David and stylish Dr. Hampton watched me catwalk down the hall, I focused on doing my best, being a good student of walking. I took slow, deliberate, wide steps. I focused on lifting my toes, which refused to flex upward on their own. *Concentrate, Andrea.*

Back on the exam table, Dr. Hampton asked me to sit with my hands on my knees, palms flat, and to then turn both over as fast as possible. Back and forth, a patty-cake game with myself. My patty-cake, however, was way too slow. No matter how hard I concentrated on speeding it up, I couldn't. Tears pricked at my eyes. *Try harder. Just try harder, Andrea.*

Dr. Hampton scheduled a variety of blood tests to rule out conditions like Lyme disease and vitamin deficiency. She wrote a prescription for four MRIs to capture images from my brain and down my spine. She scheduled a nerve conduction study and an electromyography (EMG) test that could be done in their office, the next day. I appreciated something that could get checked off quickly.

As she walked toward the door, she said, "The EMG is uncomfortable, but you can always tell the doctor to turn it down."

"Turn what down?" I asked.

"The electric current," she said, closing the door.

◦◦◦

The next day, I stripped down to my bra and underwear for the EMG test. I tried to arrange the paper sheet more for warmth than modesty. I was freezing.

Dr. Anderson, the physician administering the EMG, entered the room. He explained that an EMG measured muscle response or electrical activity in response to the nerve's stimulation of the muscle. The test would be used to detect neuromuscular abnormalities in the lower motor neurons. *Neuromuscular abnormalities?*

He explained that he would ask me to flex a muscle, then stick a needle (!) into the muscle for several seconds. Then he would tell me to relax the muscle as he watched a computer screen attached to a machine that had sound effects.

He said we were aiming for silence once I let the muscle relax.

I didn't like the sound of this. Not for even a second. *Wait, what?* His instructions caught me completely off guard.

I was suddenly sweating and cold at the same time. *It's okay,* I told myself. *It will be fine.*

"Are you ready?" he asked.

I nodded.

Dr. Anderson started with the top of my foot. He told me to flex my foot upward. I did. He then plunged a needle into my skin. I gasped. *Holy mother of . . .*

A loud, scratchy, crackly sound filled the room—like a ham radio operator trying to tune in to a faraway station. Dr. Anderson counted down from ten. The needle remained buried in the top of my foot. I looked away.

After ten seconds, he told me to relax. I released my foot (and the breath I had been holding).

The crackly noise immediately dissipated. Just a couple of pings. *Seriously, who comes up with this bullshit?*

I closed my eyes and decided to go someplace else in my mind. Unsure how many more needles would be stuck into my body, I needed an escape.

I chose the memory of Monterrico, Guatemala, and the night I spent sleeping in a hammock on its black-sand beach. I was twenty, a junior in college studying abroad for the semester—the longest time I had ever been on my own.

Sleeping outdoors in a far-off country with an active volcano nearby was definitely the wildest thing I'd ever done. I felt grown-up, sexy, and free—and also very much like a scared little girl. The gentle swaying of the hammock combined with the soothing lapping of the waves made me sleepy, but the moon was too bright on the inside of my eyelids when I closed them.

Eventually, I decided this was a once-in-a-lifetime kind of night. I got up quietly so as not to disturb my friend Kate in the hammock next to me. I walked out onto the sand alone and sat for hours, hugging my knees, watching the moonlight dancing on the waves, staring out at the infinite mysteries of the ocean.

"If a therapist ever tells me to go to my happy place, this is it," I joked to Kate the next morning.

Boy, I never imagined this needle-in-the-foot-and-everywhere-else scenario.

"Again," Dr. Anderson said, before plunging another needle into my body, a shoulder this time.

By this point, I had lost track of how many times he jammed a needle into my muscles. But it was a lot. He had moved up my body slowly: calves, thighs, stomach, back, even the crooks of my thumbs. He fiddled with dials, seemingly trying to reach aliens through the crackling sounds that commenced with each needle stick.

I was miserable. How long could I endure this?

"Relax, you have to relax," he said over and over again. "Make the noise go away." *I'd do anything to make the noise go away.* But I refused to ask him to turn the current down, as Dr. Hampton had suggested. I would tough this out.

When we were finally done, he asked me how I felt.

"I don't think I'll ever be able to look at torture scenes in movies the same way again," I said, rubbing my arm, picturing the electrocution scene from *Taken*.

He laughed, and then was a little serious. "I've been told it's like something out of Guantanamo—by people who would know." This was Washington, DC, after all.

Dr. Anderson continued. "I am relieved, though. You passed. With your symptoms, when you came in here, I was worried."

"What were you worried about?" I asked.

"Oh, um, well, I think you need to talk to Dr. Hampton about that," he said. "I just mean, um, I think some big possibilities can be ruled out."

❧

"He said *what?*" David practically yelled when I called him from the safety of the busy street outside. "How could he not tell you what the results were?"

"I don't know," I said. "What's the big deal? The test is over. And whatever it was, Dr. Anderson said it was ruled *out*."

"It's just unprofessional," David snapped.

A couple weeks after the EMG test, I began reading *I Remember Running*, a memoir by Darcy Wakefield. She was diagnosed with ALS in her mid-thirties.

The painful test that led to her diagnosis sounded awfully familiar. *Thank God I don't have ALS*, I thought. But still, it hit a little too close to home.

I put the book away.

Pre-diagnosis: February 2014

Dr. Hampton was stumped.

The bloodwork, four MRIs, nerve conduction study, and EMG all came back normal. *Normal. Nothing about what is going on with me is freaking normal.*

"Most people have shadows on their MRIs that I have to explain away," she said. "You don't even have that. Your brain is perfect."

Based on the tests, she gave us the list of what was ruled out: multiple sclerosis, tumors, Lyme disease, many autoimmune disorders, a variety of vitamin deficiencies, and at least ten other conditions.

And yes, she confirmed that the clean EMG ruled out ALS.

We had the list of "not this," but no idea of the "possibly this." As a result, Dr. Hampton ordered a new round of tests, including a spinal tap and CT scan. She gave me the names of three movement disorder specialists at university hospitals.

"Is that a real thing? A 'movement disorder specialist'?" I asked, laughing a bit. Sounded like a made-up title, like a Disney Imagineer.

She arched a perfect eyebrow at me. "Yes, it's a real discipline. A subspecialty dealing with more rare neurological conditions. Like Parkinson's." *Oh. Okay, I'm a jerk.*

Dr. Hampton continued. "Call them all and go to the one who can see you the soonest. They have crazy waitlists. At least four to six months."

My mouth dropped open. *Four to six months without any clue what is going on with me?*

"Call them every week. You must be annoying about it. They must know your name. Make them sick of you. If they know your name and they're sick of you calling and someone cancels, boom, you're in."

I looked at David and shook my head, disappointed and bewildered. *Crazy.*

❧

With new appointments scheduled three, four, and five months out and a calendar reminder set for every Tuesday at 10 A.M. to call and pester the front desk staff at the movement disorder specialists' offices, I found myself looking forward to the spinal tap and CT scan. I didn't fear the pain anymore; I feared the stagnation of not knowing, of no progress. I needed forward movement toward some sort of answer. The sooner I got a diagnosis, the sooner we could fix it and get on with starting a family.

I scheduled a second opinion appointment with Dr. Kendall in Philadelphia, a neurologist recommended by Dr. Dave.

The appointment with Dr. Kendall was scheduled for the day after the spinal tap. My plan was to go solo to the spinal tap appointment in DC, then hop on a train to Philly, where I would stay the night with my in-laws before Dr. Kendall's appointment.

I had convinced David he didn't need to attend all the medical appointments with me—since there appeared to be no end in sight. As a junior attorney in a large DC law firm, he was slammed with work and under pressure to bill hours, impress partners, and attend happy hours. All of which resulted in David often leaving the office at midnight. The last thing I wanted to do was add to his stress.

Besides, no one told me that my spinal-tap-plus-train-ride plan was a terrible idea.

❧

The official name for a spinal tap is a lumbar puncture.

The goal of the procedure is to collect cerebellar spinal fluid (CSF) for analysis. CSF is the fluid that suspends the gray matter of our brains inside our skulls. To extract it, the doctor inserts a huge needle into the spinal canal—like tapping sap from a tree to make maple syrup.

Strapped to a table and inverted so my legs were above my head, I started to care very much after all whether the procedure would hurt. But thanks to the local anesthesia applied to the spot on my spine where the needle was inserted, I felt no pain. The whole procedure only took a few minutes.

"Who came with you, dear?" asked the nurse.

"No one," I said. "Is that a problem?"

"Hmm," she said. "Well, you need to lie flat for the next twenty-four hours at least."

"What?" I squeaked, still upside down. "I'm supposed to take a train to Philly to get to another doctor's appointment tomorrow."

She explained that my body would need a few days to regenerate the fluid drained out for analysis. If I was sitting up or standing, gravity would prevent the fluid from reaching my brain and I would end up with a horrible headache.

So much for the plan to minimize disruptions to David's work.

David fetched me from the stretcher in the ICU recovery area and cradled my head in his lap on the cab ride home. I was a little woozy but generally okay, I assured David, as he returned to work. The hardest part was me later trying to hail a cab to Union Station with my head cocked sideways—the best angle I could manage.

On the crowded train headed to Philly, I stretched out across two seats. I put on dark sunglasses and headphones, and lay with my head flat on the seat, swaddled by my down puffy coat. I tried to make myself look sufficiently unapproachable while also avoiding the annoyed looks from fellow passengers.

Dr. Dave picked me up from 30th Street Station. I lay down in the back seat all the way to David's childhood home. I stared up at the dark outline of passing treetops while being chauffeured—a visual perspective I hadn't seen since my own childhood.

Up to that point, I had been doing well at squashing my emotions, staying neutral. I treated the whole diagnosis chasing like a work project, maybe even a triathlon. *Stay organized and know what the next step is, but don't get too far ahead of yourself. Just be patient and work the problem in front of you. Above all, don't freak out. No need to worry until there's a reason to worry.*

I sounded very calm inside my head—and outside, too. Maybe I *had* learned a thing or two.

I was healthy, after all. Every bizarre medical test and doctor to date had confirmed it. In fact, the only thing making me sick at that point *was* one of the bizarre tests. Tight hamstrings and not being able to play patty-cake is not a disease. We just needed to figure out what was going on, fix it, and move on. Thanks to triathlon training, I was in the best shape of my life.

The morning after the spinal tap, I felt worse. Every time I sat up in bed, my head pounded with a sickening headache. When I lay down, the headache evaporated. Caffeine was supposed to help, so I downed soda after soda through a straw while lying flat on my back.

Still, I managed to work lying on my back. I conducted a few calls before Dr. Dave and I set out for Dr. Kendall's. I look back now and wonder what could have been so important that I refused to call in sick.

The slow walk from the bedroom caused such vicious nausea that I almost threw up. I slumped flat in the back seat of the car, and then on a loveseat in the doctor's waiting room, dictating to my father-in-law what to write on the intake forms as I stared at the ceiling.

Dr. Kendall proved to be a kindly old doctor with just the right mix of pleasantries and efficiency. His tests were similar to Dr. Hampton's.

"You're really strong," he said more than once during the exam.

I laughed. "Well, I should be. I just did a 70-mile triathlon." *Well, five months ago.*

He popped my heel with the palm of his hand. With the quick strike, my leg started shaking uncontrollably. I forgot about my aching head for a moment and looked up at him, surprised.

"Clonus," he said.

He explained that clonus happens when the neurological signal to move a specific body part doesn't reach its intended target. The signal, instead, bounces around. So that weird, inexplicable *thing* that had been happening for months on Metro escalators and when I tried to shave my legs on the side of the bathtub actually had a name. I mentally added *clonus* to my vocabulary, alongside *foot drop*, the official term for constantly feeling like I was tripping over my toes. I was comforted to pick up another clue; however, these pearls of wisdom from neurological oracles were being dispensed far too slowly.

By the time he finished his tests, my dizziness was astounding. Bright spots appeared and my vision blurred. The metallic taste of nausea flooded my mouth. My brain throbbed from the lack of spinal fluid.

As Dr. Dave and I settled into Dr. Kendall's office around the enormous oak desk, I slumped as low as possible to minimize the angle and rate of spinal fluid draining away from my thirsty brain.

My brain felt like a cartoon goldfish—flopping at the bottom of the dry bowl of my skull, gasping and wheezing its last breaths as Dr. Kendall traded medical theories with my father-in-law.

"Would you like to lie down?" Dr. Kendall asked me.

"More than anything," I sighed. The cartoon goldfish for a brain nodded also.

They moved chairs around the cramped office, and I curled up on the floor at the base of the huge desk. The conversation continued over my head, literally and figuratively. Once I was lying down, the spinal fluid rushed in, saving the cartoon goldfish brain from its certain demise.

Dr. Kendall didn't have any answers, but offered to call a colleague he described as the best diagnostician on the East Coast. He also called in a prescription for a "blood patch," an injection to seal the spinal tap injection site—to prevent spinal fluid from continuing to leak from the puncture point.

"You'll feel better within a half hour after the injection," he promised. I was amazed and then annoyed. *Who comes up with this stuff? And why is this the first time anyone is mentioning it?*

Before we left, I asked one question I did not want to ask.

"We're supposed to go to Hawaii on vacation in two weeks for my parents' fiftieth anniversary," I said, still lying sideways.

Dr. Kendall looked at me. "I wouldn't recommend it," he said.

"What? Why?" I squealed.

Without thinking, I jerked my head up so I could see him over the edge of the desk. The cartoon goldfish brain, in that moment, leapt clear out of the bowl. I crumpled back to the carpet.

"You're a serious fall risk. Why take unnecessary chances?"

At that moment, I started to realize how small my world was about to become.

I was now the goldfish.

"You gotta remember, he's over seventy years old," Dr. Dave said to me on the ride home. "Risk to him looks a lot different than risk to you."

In the end, I came to the same conclusion. I was just as much of a fall risk in DC as I was on the Big Island of Hawaii.

Two weeks later, across the country, every sunset I watched, every humpback whale breach I glimpsed in the wide-open Pacific, every night spent staring up at the endless field of stars brought Dr. Kendall's words back to me. *Why take chances?* Because that's where the beauty of life is.

CHAPTER 6

A GUST OF WIND

Pre-diagnosis: March 2014

The moment I realized I could no longer walk on my own came as I lay in the middle of the street, staring up at the headlights from oncoming cars.

Spring that year had no interest in a graceful cherry-blossom reveal. Working from a coffee shop one afternoon, I watched out the window as menacing dark clouds took over the first mild, blue-sky day DC had seen in months. When the wind started whipping the bare branches of the trees, I packed up to walk the five blocks home. (Later, I learned these wind gusts had topped sixty miles an hour.)

My legs were heavy and stiff as I walked, something I noticed happening more often, especially after sitting for any length of time. *Lift your toes, lift your toes* became my walking mantra. The temperature had dropped by at least twenty degrees. I shivered in the light sweater I'd been so excited to put on that morning.

As I crossed an intersection, a strong gust of wind funneled between the office buildings. The wind grabbed me and I went sprawling—gashing my thumb on the pavement, smashing the phone in my hand, tearing a hole in the knee of my jeans.

I looked up to see the headlights of oncoming cars waiting for the light to turn. I tried to gather myself quickly and jump up from the pavement, but I was frozen, pinned to the ground. The messenger bag slung over my shoulder was like a cinder block, weighing me down.

Before I had time to panic, I felt myself being hoisted up from behind.

"Oh, Miss," said a voice. "Let me help you. Let's go, quickly!"

Dumbly, I nodded, trying to grasp what happened. *My phone! I'm bleeding! Did a gust of wind really just knock me over?* (I hate to admit the order in which those thoughts occurred.)

After sputtering my thanks and protesting that *I am fine, really*, the stranger helped me into a cab for the four blocks home.

The episode scared me into buying a Hurrycane from As Seen On TV. In addition to appreciating a good pun, I loved the ingenuity of the cane's design. A collapsible, tent-like pole with a stretchy nylon cord inside, the Hurrycane folded up nicely so I could hide it under my desk at work or the bar at happy hour. When I was ready to go, I simply lifted the Hurrycane handle, let it unfurl, and all four segments snapped together smartly.

The carefree days of the Hurrycane were short-lived, though.

Only two months later, I was too unstable for its little swiveling base. Walking began to require vigilant concentration. It wasn't just my toes anymore—my entire body and balance was off-kilter. If my attention wandered for an instant—*boom!* I was on the floor.

I upgraded to a giant four-footed cane. But the next day, even the behemoth cane couldn't keep me from falling through the closing doors of a Metro train during my morning commute. I was dragged up to my feet by a stranger—again.

I sat down in the Metro seat kindly vacated for me, in a train car that suddenly seemed much too silent for rush hour. I put on my sunglasses—even though the train was still underground—and cried.

⌘

The best diagnostician on the East Coast, Dr. Jensen, thought I was suffering from stiff person syndrome (SPS), a bizarre neurological condition that causes a person's muscles to all freeze at once and the poor person then topples over like a statue.

Apparently, Dr. Jensen formulated that theory after the first sentence I spoke.

"How do you feel?" she asked me as we walked down the hall.

"Stiff," I said, concentrating on walking without tripping.

After her exam, she told me about SPS.

"I can usually figure out someone's condition by the first thing they say," she said. She sent me home with a prescription for a rare blood test that cost a thousand dollars and wasn't covered by insurance.

The results came back negative.

"I'm not sure why she thought you had stiff person syndrome," said Dr. Smith, the movement disorder specialist I finally saw in April, three months after Dr. Hampton told me to pester the front desk with weekly calls. "Your muscles don't stiffen up all at the same time."

I shrugged, agitated. *You guys are supposed to be the experts.*

"You need to understand that there aren't any definitive tests for these conditions," Dr. Smith told David and me. "At this point, it's all process of elimination and matching up symptoms. That's what makes diagnosing a rare disease so challenging."

"There's a doctor I want you to see," said Dr. Smith. "Dr. Caustik is a specialist in ALS and something called primary lateral sclerosis (PLS)."

He continued. "Now, I don't want you to worry about this," he said. "PLS is a far-distant cousin of ALS, and ALS has already been ruled out."

But the internet told us there was plenty of reason to worry.

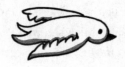

CHAPTER 7

THE PROBABLE
DIAGNOSIS

Pre-diagnosis: March 2014

The middle of a health crisis is probably a horrible time to buy a house. But David and I were grasping for something stable to hold on to during the swirling uncertainty. A house provided a very literal anchor for us.

We decided to buy one.

On the best days, the house proved that we were moving ahead with our lives, come what may on the medical front.

On the worst days, we pretended our plans of having a family were not completely derailed. Most days, though, a new house was just a welcome distraction. Something to look forward to.

I loved our downtown DC apartment. Sometimes I stayed awake at night looking out our bedroom window, entranced by the view: the majestic, illuminated Greek columns and rippled glass roof of the National Portrait Gallery. Beyond it, the Washington Monument—iconic, welcoming, and austere all at once. My eyes soaked in the scene; I wanted to remember it forever.

But it was only *inside* our apartment that I felt safe. The bustling Chinatown street life I'd loved as an urban planner was now far too intimidating. Too treacherous. Too full of uneven brick sidewalks. Too full of people walking fast with their heads buried in their phones, certainly not expecting to run into a thirty-three-year-old walking slowly with a four-footed cane. The radius around our apartment that I was willing to walk was shrinking—first to a few blocks, then to a block, then to just businesses on our side of the street so I didn't have to cross an intersection.

This was the opposite of the freedom I'd felt when we initially moved downtown. That's when we had achieved every city planner's dream by selling our car. I loved that we were saving money and the environment. Healthier, too, since we could walk or bike everywhere or opt for transit if the weather was bad. Sustainable idealism at its finest.

Now we made a game of renting a carshare and scouting open houses every weekend in DC neighborhoods and in the Maryland and Virginia suburbs. Did we want a rowhouse in the revitalizing Petworth corridor? A cute bungalow in Takoma Park?

Imagining each possible future was exciting, but every potential home forced us to stop and consider our reality. *What if it gets to the point I can no longer climb stairs? We should find a place with a bedroom on the first floor. Maybe we could craft a bedroom out of this dining room if we had to . . .*

We found a quirky ranch in Silver Spring, Maryland, only a quarter mile from the Forest Glen Metro train station. According to the neighbors, the owners in the 1970s were sisters who didn't like each other very much. So even though it looked like a modest one-story from the front, the sisters tacked on an addition to the back of the house and finished off the basement, resulting in three levels with several living spaces and bedrooms to serve as buffers between them. For us, the funky trilevel layout created flexibility to adapt to changes in our situation. Plenty of room for multiple kids, but if stairs ever became too difficult, the main floor had access to every room I needed.

Although our plan was to commute to work via the Metro, within a week it became obvious that we would still need a car for the suburbs. We debated heading straight to the minivan for kids or—*ugh*—a wheelchair. We settled on a used Subaru wagon with good trade-in value.

In the end, I walked to the Metro exactly once. Too many driveway curb cuts and too many uneven sidewalks. I didn't want to get knocked over by the rush of commuters either. The city I'd loved to run around and wander through now felt utterly hostile and unforgiving. I traded the walkable, transit-friendly, urban excitement of DC for the automobile-centric sprawl of the suburbs. Oh, the irony.

At that point, I was alone.

No, that wasn't right. I *felt* alone. I had David, and he had me. But we were spinning in circles around my condition—whatever it was. We were alone together.

I needed to be open about my struggle with more than just my inner circle. I put all the words and feelings on my personal blog.

The outpouring of support we received, from heartfelt emails and texts to bouquets of flowers, convinced me that speaking up was the right decision. We didn't need help per se; we just needed to feel less alone.

However, the downside of going public with this type of news? Everyone (and I mean everyone) had a theory about what *it* was. Of what I needed to get well: mostly prayer, gingko biloba, and local honey, it seemed.

Mom's coworker told her that chemicals used as fire retardant in bed sheets had been linked to neurological conditions. Mom began an intense research crusade and subsequent email chain about this theory. Lucky for me, I had the wrong sheets.

Mom then emailed a triathlete who was diagnosed with chronic lymphocytic leukemia. We had no overlapping symptoms, mind you, but Mom hoped he could recommend a doctor with experience treating athletes. Her outreach was painful in its earnest awkwardness, and I was overwhelmed enough without her "help." I had a full-time job, coupled with numerous medical appointments and packing for our move to the new house. To say nothing of the free-floating undercurrent of anxiety about how and why my body was betraying me. I needed help. But I needed *real* help. There was nothing Mom could do from two states away.

I desperately needed her to work smarter, not harder. But that was not our family's way.

Eventually, I gave her a list of productive things to do. The new list, such as researching acupuncture and looking for a nutritionist who worked in an integrative medicine practice, was a better use of everyone's time. David also suggested that she (quietly) make a list of all the conditions people told her about, or that she read about on the internet, and promised to inquire about everything on the list at my next doctor's appointment.

Predictably, she felt bad.

Predictably, I felt guilty for making her feel bad.

That *was* our family's way.

Pre-diagnosis: May 2014

Two weeks after closing on the house, David and I headed out of town to see yet another neurologist—the one specializing in ALS and PLS—Dr. Caustik. David's parents drove down for the day, sensing we were close to getting some answers.

From the moment my eyes opened that morning, I was frazzled.

My in-laws arrived at our hotel room to find papers spread all over the bed. I had frantically rearranged my orange medical notebook and filled out yet another stack of new patient paperwork. I was mad at myself for waiting until the last minute, then impatient I couldn't write faster. David and his mom took over handwriting duties, while I dictated answers and put my notebook back together. *Okay, let's go. Appointment at noon. We gotta go now.*

As the four of us piled into the hallway, my foot caught on the doorjamb.

I fell face first onto the rough carpet, which greeted me with a smashed lip and rug burns on my cheek and knuckles. Tears welled, but we were cutting it so close that I wiped them away, saying "I'm fine, I'm fine!" before anyone could protest or delay us further.

Dr. Dave guided me out to the car. David went to the hotel front desk to grab ice for my battered face.

We rushed into the hospital. I was barely holding it together. I attempted to check in at the electronic kiosk on the Neurology floor. The first message I read on the screen: "Please check in 30 minutes before your appointment." The appointment was at noon. The time? 11:55.

Before I could stop myself, a loud wail escaped my throat. I just flat out lost my composure. The stress, the fall, my failure as a model patient, a model daughter, a model wife. It was just too much. I was sobbing. *I try so hard and yet here we are. It's all crumbling down. My health, my body, my career, my future. No matter what I've achieved, what I've been through—it doesn't matter. I had one simple thing to do—show up on time—and I failed.*

My in-laws crept away to give us some space. David took my hand and led me to a chair, talking softly. I took ragged breaths. I pressed the flimsy plastic cup of hotel ice to my swollen lip, as he walked over to speak with the receptionist. He walked back to me smiling.

"Everything is fine," he said. "No one gets here a half hour early. Don't worry."

I nodded, closed my eyes, and took a deep breath. *I still feel like I am failing.*

⁓

Dr. Caustik was my kind of neurologist—friendly and efficient. And she liked my organized orange notebook. Her exam was quick, but when she asked questions, she really listened to our answers.

"Do you think your voice has been affected?" she asked.

David piped up. "I think her voice has slowed down. I noticed it when listening to her voicemail." I turned toward him in surprise.

Dr. Caustik nodded. "Can you play it?"

David dialed my number, placing the phone on speaker mode. In a few seconds, we heard my chirpy voice rattle off: "You-have-reached-Andrea-Lytle-Peet-I'm-sorry-I-missed-your-call-please-leave-your-name-number-and-message-at-the-beep-and-I-will-get-back-to-you-as-soon-as-possible-thanks-and-have-a-great-day." All in one breath. *Shit. He's right.*

"That's called dysarthria," Dr. Caustik said. "Now, have you noticed uncontrollable laughing or crying?"

We all stared at her. *You mean like in your waiting room fifteen minutes ago?*

Seeing our faces, she said, "That's called pseudobulbar effect."

"What about fasciculations?" she asked. When I looked at her blankly, she clarified. "Do you have any muscle twitching?"

I shook my head. "Good, good," she said. (Of course, immediately after the appointment, I started noticing the twitching. A brief fluttering in my thigh muscle, a ping in my shoulder. *Add it to the list of ways I'm falling apart.*)

Dr. Caustik went on to deliver the clearest neurological explanation to date about what was happening to my body.

"For any muscle in your body to move, two main nerve connections must happen. First, when you think, 'I want to take a step,' your brain sends the message to your spinal cord through the *upper* motor neurons. The spinal cord then signals the appropriate muscles to flex via the *lower* motor neurons, long fibers that extend all the way to your glutes, thighs, knees, ankles, and toes. The signaling process is so rapid that it seems instantaneous and unconscious—you're just walking."

I had not understood how truly magnificent the human body was until that moment.

ALS is diagnosed when *both* the upper and lower motor neurons are compromised, but the effect on the lower motor neurons is what makes ALS deadly. The EMG—those nasty needles stuck into my muscles—tested the lower motor neurons. *But I passed!*

As a result, Dr. Caustik was looking toward primary lateral sclerosis (PLS) as my possible diagnosis. PLS only affects the upper motor neurons.

With PLS, the message delivery is slow between the brain and the spinal cord, resulting in slow speech, slow handwriting, slow walking, tight muscles, being startled easily, and overall weakness—which mirrored my symptoms. Although it takes longer for the messages to get to the muscles, they can still respond. PLS is not considered life *shortening*, even though it is progressive and many people end up in wheelchairs.

"Don't get excited," she warned as she finished her explanation. "Most doctors won't diagnose PLS for at least two years because sometimes the upper motor neuron symptoms emerge before the lower. And I still want to do my own EMG so we have a baseline on the lower motor neurons."

The prospect of being stabbed with needles again did not faze me. I had my family with me, and I'd aced that wretched test only five months before.

Best of all, we might finally have our answer.

❦

By the time we took a break so the room could be prepped for the EMG, it was almost two in the afternoon.

David had a conference call scheduled for work—an important one.

"Are you sure you don't need me to stay?" he asked worriedly, but I waved him off. I knew the call was important, and really, my copious medical appointments had already taken up so much time. His mom could stay with me.

He said, "I love you so much. I'll be back as soon as I can." He kissed me, then left with Dr. Dave to take the call from the car in the parking deck.

I undressed down to my underwear and lay down on the table, covering myself with the paper-thin sheet. Dr. Caustik walked in holding my orange notebook.

"Wow, I'll say your last EMG was thorough," she said. I felt vindicated. I knew that damn test was horrible.

"Okay, here we go. Flex." I felt the needle pierce my skin and tear through my ankle muscle. The scratchy, crackly, ham radio noise again. I sighed and closed my eyes. *Here we go again.*

For a while, Dr. Caustik said nothing except "flex" and "relax." I slammed my eyes tight, concentrating on breathing evenly and willing the noise to go away. *Please, please, please end this nightmare. A life in a wheelchair will be okay. But just let me pass this test again.*

"It's actually a good thing this is taking so long," she said eventually. My eyes flew open. "Some people, I stick the needle in and I know immediately. But with you, I'm really having to look."

"Take all the time you need," I said. I closed my eyes again and went back to bargaining with the universe. *Please, please, please.*

After what seemed like an hour, Dr. Caustik sat back in her chair. "Okay, we're done. You can get dressed and we'll discuss."

⁓

David and Dr. Dave had not returned, but Dr. Caustik was prepared to deliver her diagnosis.

Suddenly, I needed David—heck, both Davids—in the room. But I had my mother-in-law. It was okay. *I am okay.*

Dr. Caustik cleared her throat and launched into the criteria for a diagnosis of ALS: the El Escorial scale.

Unlike her clear-as-day explanation of the difference between ALS and PLS, I was not following her words. I needed a minute. *El Escorial?*

According to the El Escorial criteria, an ALS diagnosis requires the following:

- Signs of degeneration of *lower motor neuron* by the EMG testing;
- Signs of degeneration of *upper motor neurons* by clinical examination of things like speech, overall weakness; and
- Progressive spread of signs within a region to other regions of the body.

ALS. El Escorial? ALS. El Escorial? ALS. El Escorial?

I still couldn't follow the words Dr. Caustik spoke. Mostly because my brain jammed every time she said "ALS."

"Uh-huh, uh-huh," I said at all the seemingly appropriate moments.

"So there is involvement in your arms and legs. It's very slight, but it's there," she said.

"Uh-huh," I said. Wait, what?

"So, what questions do you have for me?" she asked.

I had all the questions, and none of them at the same time. At that point, I supposed there was only one question. I swallowed hard and looked past her eyes.

"Are you saying I have ALS?" my voice was a mere whisper. I was trying desperately not to cry.

She paused. "Well, you don't meet the full criteria for definite ALS."

I blinked. *El Escorial?*

Dr. Caustik continued. "For patients who don't meet the *full criteria* for ALS, we have a category called 'probable ALS,' which in reality . . ." She trailed off for a split second, then picked back up. "What is the point of a diagnosis? If the point of a diagnosis is to get you necessary resources and get you into clinical trials, then we can do that now."

What is the point of a diagnosis? What is the point??

David and Dr. Dave returned, and I asked Dr. Caustik to repeat the news for them. Hoping maybe I would hear something new, something that made sense. But her explanation was like a slippery fish that I couldn't quite grasp. And anyway, it was getting harder to focus on anything besides my rumbling stomach.

I looked at David. He looked at me, concerned and a bit puzzled. But mostly he looked like he wanted to get out of there. I did too. Dr. Dave and my mother-in-law were quiet, concerned looks on their faces.

I repeated in my head. *Probable ALS. I probably have ALS.*

Looking back, Dr. Caustik could have saved us months of confusion, frustration, and pain if she had left the medical jargon behind and just told us in words we could understand.

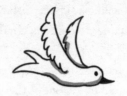

CHAPTER 8

'TIL DEATH
DO US PART

Purgatory: May 2014

David and I weren't sure what to do with this news of probable ALS.

We sat on the hotel room bed. We turned over and over what Dr. Caustik had said, trying to make sense of it. We ate takeout Thai. And finally, as Dr. Caustik suggested, we scheduled a visit to the ALS Clinic for mid-June. *At least there is a plan. I appreciate a plan.*

We did not research anything on the internet (for once). We discussed if we could modify our new house for a wheelchair. Whether we could afford the house at all with only David's salary.

Every topic that evening was laced with two weird words: *Probable. Hope.*

Hope was worse than *probable.*

Hope ping-ponged between us like a cruel joke. I would say something. There would be a pause, and David would send a volley back.

I hope the ALS Clinic has some answers.

I hope we can afford the house with all these things we'll need.

I hope I can keep working.

I hope that probable ALS isn't ALS.

Probable ALS? Still a chance of no ALS, right? Like the weather? Probable rain—sometimes means no rain?

Eventually, we ran out of safe topics. Our conversation trailed off. Just that morning, I had face-planted in the hotel hallway; it felt like months ago. I had hoped for answers today. *Be careful what you wish for.* I got answers, but none of them clear. *Hope. Answers. Probable.*

We numbed ourselves with the television and a late-night show. The show featured a comedian, but I couldn't laugh. I wondered if I'd ever laugh again.

At some point, we fell asleep with the lights on. I slept fitfully all night, dreaming my go-to stress dream. Wedding planning. Now *that* was its own sort of nightmare.

Pre-pre-pre-pre-diagnosis: Our Wedding, June 2009

Five years earlier, our wedding had been beautiful and fun. Everyone said so, even past the point of being polite. I was glad, considering I nearly destroyed myself planning it.

David proposed two years before our wedding, creating an end date for our long-distance relationship. I would spend two years in Atlanta for grad school, then we would get married. Afterward, I would join David in DC for his third year of law school.

At first, wedding planning provided a welcome distraction from schoolwork and missing David. I used my free time to research and obsess over every detail. I imagined all the centerpieces and wedding favors I would create by hand. Not that I am one of those crafty people. But what I lack in craftiness, I make up for in hard work.

The wedding industry, of course, was willing to conspire with my obsession. *Say Yes to the Dress* and *My Big Fat American Gypsy Wedding* and *Bridezillas*—I watched all the bridal reality TV shows. I gobbled up every wedding magazine I could find.

"Your wedding dress is the most important, most photographed piece of clothing you'll ever own," warned the wedding shows. *50 Mistakes Every Bride Makes*, cautioned the magazines.

I knew I was being suckered by the marketing, but I was already drunk on champagne flutes of bride hysteria.

Wedding Dress Shopping Day arrived. I marched with purpose and knowledge into the boutique flanked by Mom and Cathy, my matron of honor. I tried on one white dress after another, waiting for the blissful moment of transcendence (as seen on TV). That special moment I found "the" dress. The moment the tears would flow and my Mom and I would gasp in stereo.

I waited. For the moment I would *know*.

By late afternoon, my tears were of frustration and low blood sugar. My petite frame looked *fine* in all the dresses, but the salesperson had gotten in my head with a terrifying question:

"Who do you want to *be* on your wedding day?"

I did not have an answer for her. A sexy bride? A glamorous bride? A princess bride? (Okay, I never wanted to be a princess bride.) The three of us left the store after five hours, dejected.

After food and a good night's sleep, I had the answer. I wanted to look like myself. And so, with considerably less zeal and fanfare, Mom and I drove to an underwhelming bridal emporium. I picked a dress with a customizable ribbon. I looked pretty in that pretty white dress. I looked like myself.

I wish I could say that the experience taught me a lesson—that I fought the wedding-industry hysteria hype and won—but that would be a lie. I was deeply disappointed in myself and stuck in bridal purgatory: I could neither cry spontaneous tears of joy nor convince my bride-TV brain that it was just a dress.

Mostly, I ruined the quintessential mother-daughter experience by pushing too hard. *I always push too hard.*

The planning trudged on like a sled I pushed from behind.

In the throes of planning the most important—and of course, *happiest*—day of my life, I just felt like I was failing. I succeeded only at spreading my misery to everyone else, which added a heavy stack of guilt to my wedding planning sled.

Mom got the worst of my misery. The fantasy of the wedding had long evaporated. The wedding was now a difficult job, and I, its jaded project manager. Mom was the employee who took the brunt of my disgruntlement.

David, meanwhile, was putting in long hours as a second-year summer associate at a DC law firm. These positions often led to full-time offers after graduation, so he was doing a great job at *that job*. But he wasn't much help with the wedding job (*ahem*, the one I had created). Truthfully, David's distance from Wedding HQ was probably the safest arrangement for our upcoming marriage.

But I missed his calming presence.

Instead, I tested the limits of Mom's patience, which I had previously assumed was infinite. She put up with my snarky remarks, mini tantrums, and eye rolls. One day, I found her limit.

"I don't know what to do with you! Everything I say is wrong," she said to me, exasperated.

We have never agreed on anything related to décor, style, or standards of bedroom cleanliness. So, of course, we didn't agree on wedding details. Her style was too fussy, too matchy-matchy; her ways too methodical and slow. I was modern in my choices; too busy, efficient, and impatient to care about the things she fretted over.

Mostly, I dismissed her suggestions out of principle—or perhaps habit. *Don't you know me at all?*

Her words should have shaken some sense into me, but I had sealed myself off inside a hornet's nest of panic about the wedding and self-loathing about how I was handling the stress. No way could I hear her over the angry buzzing.

Three days before the wedding, I called Mom from the hardware store—what I was doing there, I can't remember. The meltdown was intense.

"I just can't do it anymore!" I wailed into my cell phone.

"Come on back home. We can talk about it when you get here," she said evenly. Her mask of infinite patience had been restored.

❦

In the end, I survived the happiest day of my life.

Our wedding was beautiful and full of personal touches, just as I planned. But as I look through our wedding album, photos of me reveal emptiness behind my eyes. I was posing for the camera like a good bride should.

There is one photo I love, however.

Snapped in the moment I first saw David as I walked down the aisle, those tears of joy were real.

Although I agonized over every single detail of the wedding, I never once questioned the marriage. At least that part I got absolutely right.

Myrtle Beach: May 2014

Speaking of weddings. Two days after the probable ALS diagnosis, David and I went to a friend's wedding.

In case you were wondering, going to a wedding is the absolute worst thing you can do after you have been (probably) diagnosed with a certainly terminal illness. A stupid thing to do, really.

Of course, David knew this from the outset. He asked me three times if we could cancel.

I told him—each time—that no, we couldn't. We had to attend.

The bride's parents and my parents had been friends for forty years—almost since the first day my parents arrived in Raleigh. When the bride's father discovered that Andy and Sandy were camping in a local park to save money, he insisted they move in with him until they found a place. Our families had spent nearly every Christmas together since. *Those* kinds of friends. Like family.

Mom and Dad picked us up from the airport in the sticky humidity of Myrtle Beach, South Carolina. The sky was overcast with saggy gray clouds, matching our moods: heavy, oppressive, dark. *A perfect day for a wedding.*

After we received the news from Dr. Caustik, David and I had called Mom and Dad immediately. But in the car two days later, they said nothing about probable ALS. Not a word.

Dad drove with a fake smile plastered across his face. Mom made inane small talk, turning around far too often to look at me.

David and I exchanged confused, annoyed glances in the back seat. *How could they not say anything?*

During the wedding, David squeezed my hand as the words "to have and to hold, in sickness and in health, 'til death do us part" were repeated by the lovely couple.

I suddenly had a headache. Those words. *Bullshit.*

Words ingrained in our culture. *Bullshit.* Words that assume a bright future. *Bullshit.* Words that distill love down into impossible, simple tropes. *Bullshit.*

At the reception, we endured endless toasts and jokes about future children, holidays and decades to come, growing old together, grandchildren and . . . and . . .

Bullshit. Bullshit! Bullshit!!

My face burned with a rage I never saw coming.

The bride was my friend. Under any other circumstances, I would have been genuinely happy for her. But any sparkle of happiness had been smothered. Buried beneath the seething lava of my anger.

I looked at the wedding attendees. All the people. All the people with lives filled with possibilities, lofty ambitions, dreams. All the people and all . . . their stupid *hope*.

All David and I could hope for? All we had to look forward to? An unraveling. A dark grief. And then, a vicious death.

I wanted to get drunk.

I wanted to dance with David, cling to him, face each other so we didn't have to face the future we wouldn't have. But being drunk meant I could not walk well. I had enough trouble doing that without wine. If walking wasn't an option, then neither was dancing.

So we just sat.

Stone cold sober, silent, miserable, staring at All The People and All Their Hope. We flatly responded to Fake Smile Dad and Small Talk Mom with one-syllable answers, until David convinced me with a series of knee squeezes under the table that we had stayed long enough to be gracious.

On the drive home, my parents insisted on stopping for hot fudge sundaes. Still no talk of probable ALS. Just Mom and Dad asking if we wanted ice cream after the torture of a wedding.

Worse than that? David and I *also* said nothing. We agreed to the ice cream.

Back at the hotel, the walls closed in. The curtains were pulled, the lights off. My head throbbed with what can only be described as an anger migraine. Suddenly, just like the moment in Dr. Caustik's waiting room, I howled.

I let it all out, tumbling deeper into grief than I ever thought possible, then realizing there was no bottom to catch me.

David tried. He reached for me, grabbed me, held me tight. The tighter he held me, the more I wailed.

After a few moments, I felt his grip loosen and his body stiffen at the same time. And he began sobbing, howling, with the same intensity I had. I flipped my arms around and pulled his head onto my shoulder.

I clutched his face as his tears soaked my skin.

We went on like this for what felt like hours. Taking turns consoling. Allowing each other to descend into the hopelessness of our lives, while the other squeezed tightly.

❧

David and I woke the next morning nursing emotional hangovers from so much crying the night before. The only thing we'd resolved is that we needed to have a real talk with my parents. Ice cream from the night before was not a bandage for the probable ALS news. Agreeing to ice cream was worse. We were all in denial.

Time to get real—all of us.

We had planned to eat brunch with Mom and Dad, but David asked them to come to our hotel room first. He texted them with one of the scariest phrases in the English language: "We need to talk."

My parents sat on one bed. We sat on the other, facing them. The curtains were still drawn, a table lamp lit between us. Interrogation style.

David took the lead. We knew I could not be trusted to handle the conversation. I was too likely to blow up in anger. The plan was for me to remain mostly silent, while David handled the hard stuff. He cleared his throat. He gave a long, measured, *lawyerly* preamble about how much we loved them and needed their support.

"Of course," Dad said. "Anything you need, you know we'll be there for you."

"You can't just say that," I interjected, then shut my mouth with a guilty sideways glance at David.

David looked at me; his eyes said *relax*.

He explained our bewilderment at their silence. No questions about probable ALS. No offers of support. No discussions of how life was going to change.

"We could see in your faces how stressed and tired you were coming off the plane," Mom said. "We just didn't want you to have to talk about it more."

The interrogation room was quiet for a beat.

"Unfortunately, we don't have the luxury of silence," David said, looking directly at her. "This is our reality now."

We continued talking, but Mom and Dad didn't understand probable ALS. David and I explained the best we could, considering we didn't really understand it either.

"Maybe you need a second opinion," Mom said. *Of course.*

I sighed. Mom doesn't trust most doctors: surgeons always want to do surgery; chiropractors are quacks; food is medicine and so is exercise. But food and exercise can't rewire the brain or connect motor neurons back to muscles. I found myself angry once again.

"Yes, we can do that," David the peacemaker said. "But we also need to consider that this neurologist is a specialist at one of the best hospitals in the country. She is in a better position to know than we are."

"But the other doctors were wrong," Mom pointed out.

I sighed again, louder. This wasn't helpful. I needed her to understand how scared I was. To understand that ALS meant death. Therefore, my diagnosis of probable ALS . . . probable death.

I needed, for the first time in a long time, for my mother to *mother* me.

"I would be happy to come up and take care of you," Dad piped up. He tried to navigate back to safer territory, as he always did.

Only that was the wrong thing to say.

"I don't want to be taken care of!" I snapped, then felt guilty immediately.

I swallowed and tried again. I tried to be calmer. "I'm thirty-three years old. I'm married. I have a full-time job. I don't want to be taken care of like a child."

"You've always been independent," Dad said, smiling. "You've been making almost all your own decisions since you were ten years old."

"She can take care of herself," David said. "At least for now. What she really needs is to feel close to you guys."

"I accepted a long time ago that we weren't close," Mom said. *A fact.*

I would have been less shocked if she'd slapped me in the face. Which of course Mom would never do. Even as a back-talking teenager, the worst I'd ever gotten was a slap *at* my wrist. My revenge? I did not talk to her for two days, one of which happened to be her birthday. I had considered it to be the worst thing I'd ever done to Mom—until this particular moment.

Her words hung in the air between us.

In those words, I flashed back to years of eye rolls and sarcastic retorts. The impact. The rift. A deep one. Mom loved me, would do anything for me, but—she was tired. She had shut down. Her patience was not infinite after all.

This was simply the moment I learned that she had given up on me. On us. On our mother-daughter relationship.

I could not move, could not speak. As if ALS had already taken over my body. Which I deserved. What kind of monster inflicts such pain on her mother? A mother whose only fault was to take whatever you dished out at her—for years?

I said I was sorry. I *was* sorry. But those were just words. *Words words words.*

The angry self-loathing buzz from my wedding returned to my ears. The buzz drowned out the conversation around the table, which had retreated to the safety of small talk—a family specialty. We have several family specialties: small talk, hard work, and *guilt.*

The guilt of their hard-earned money going toward my fancy private college, the years of my bratty teenage behavior, and the hateful bridezilla I'd become before our wedding. Mom's words from earlier repeated in my head. *I accepted a long time ago that we weren't close. Weren't close . . . Will never be close . . . Guilt guilt guilt.*

Guilty as charged.

ALS now seemed like a fitting coffin for me. I could be locked in. Controlled. Unable to inflict any more damage on the people who loved me most.

I could take my guilt and torture myself with it until it was time to die.

PART II

HOPE IS FOUND

CHAPTER 9

EMPATHY MALPRACTICE

Post–Probable ALS Diagnosis: June 2014

David and I were adrift.

We stayed indoors most of the time, wandering around in a low-grade stupor. We memorized depressing ALS facts from the internet and attempted to decipher medical journals.

The stark facts from our research belied the abysmal reality of ALS—which caused thousands of deaths per year, not to mention the cruel suffering along the way.

Where was the public outrage to this disease? ALS was like a deranged serial killer on the loose, and no one seemed to care.

Fact 1: In America, 30,000 people are living with the disease at any one time. Every ninety minutes someone is diagnosed with ALS. Every ninety minutes someone dies from it.[1]

Reality: In the time it takes to watch a movie, someone's life is ruined. And someone else's family has to bury the person they spent 24-7 taking care of for months or years, knowing that this sad moment was the only inevitable outcome.

Fact 2: Only 10 percent of cases are genetic.
Reality: Ninety percent of cases are sporadic—meaning there is no known cause.

Fact 3: The average age of ALS onset is fifty-five.
Reality: ALS can strike anyone, at any time. *Like a serial killer.*

Fact 4: What begins as a minor, strange weakness in an arm or leg usually spreads quickly. Or symptoms could start with slurred speech, known as bulbar onset.
Reality: ALS can basically attack anywhere in the body, at any time.

Fact 5: The average life expectancy after an ALS diagnosis is two to five years. Twenty percent live longer than five years; 10 percent live longer than ten years; only 5 percent survive twenty years or more.[2]
Reality: Within a few years of those first symptoms, most people with ALS are bedridden, shackled to tubes for eating and breathing—or dead.

Fact 6: All of the neurological foregoing facts occur while the person with ALS is fully conscious and fully aware, except in rare cases of associated dementia.
Reality: Everyone with ALS—(probably) me included—becomes trapped inside their failing body, forced to watch themselves die, and completely powerless to stop it.

Conclusion to All Facts: The ALS Serial Killer always wins. Also, I should quit reading the internet forever.

It felt surreal.

Tragedies like ALS happened to "others." Not to me. To friends of friends, someone featured in *People* magazine, or somebody's great-aunt. I had never even broken a bone. Just a year before, I finished triathlons. *This couldn't be happening to me.*

I missed triathlon training so much my heart hurt. I missed the glorious stress relief of a long run. After a long run you've either figured out how to move forward, or you no longer have the energy to care so damn much.

At this point, I would have given anything to be so exhausted that I could sleep soundly for a few hours. The year before, when I was stressed about time cutoffs in a race, my solution was to train more. Now, I was just restless, wound tight with anxiety, and without the release valve of a long run available to me. There were no answers to my problems.

As I drove in and out of the city, I saw runners on the sidewalks getting their doses of endorphins, vitamin D, and stress relief. Each runner made me wince with longing. I averted my eyes. If I didn't look away, the angry tears would flow. Or sometimes, I stared straight through the runners, pretending they didn't exist. *You can't fool me. You're just a mirage.* It was easier that way.

Only a year before, I was the strongest I had ever been. But all the neurologists had recommended I stop exercising until they figured out what was going on. And now? All the muscle strength I'd built was gone. And I was facing a disease that would cause my muscles to waste away. *Muscle waste. Wasted muscle.*

Dr. Caustik had cleared me to exercise. "Just don't overdo it or do anything where you might fall," she said.

My internet research taught me that a controversy existed: about whether or not people living with ALS "should" exercise. Studies of Italian professional soccer players and American football players showed statistical correlations to those athletes developing ALS later in life. Other exercise studies found no such link. All studies concluded that more studies were needed.[3] Most neurologists, reading the conflicting studies and trying to protect their patients, seemed reluctant to recommend exercise. "Don't overdo it" seemed like Dr. Caustik's way of toeing the line.

No controversy about the dangers of falling, though. I should not fall. Which meant a big fat no to cycling. And running—not that I could do that even though I desperately wanted to.

Me and my new failing body half-heartedly took to the pool and swam a couple times a week. Swimming was the last triathlon discipline available to me, but without a goal, I swam aimlessly and got bored. I was unmotivated, uninspired. *Adrift*. My technique and stamina were gone, along with my wasted muscles. *The doctors know best, right?* That's what I kept telling Mom, after all.

Twice a week, I went to the dreary National Rehabilitation Hospital (NRH) for physical therapy appointments. I battled rush hour to arrive by 8 A.M., had my hour-long appointment, and then drove home. Three hours round trip.

NRH demoralized me for reasons I couldn't pinpoint—at first. The huge, gymnasium-sized room had rows of rehab tables (mostly empty at 8 A.M.) with a few patients being stretched by their PTs, with discarded canes or wheelchairs nearby. I realized it resembled an evacuation shelter. Like when only the sick, elderly, and those who couldn't go home remained.

I wasn't elderly, but I sure felt more disabled when I walked in. I wore a race finisher T-shirt to each appointment to remind myself I was an athlete. But the more I tried to recall my races, the harder it was to believe I'd actually done them. *Was that real life?* I'd ask myself over and over. *Or is this real life?*

Also: *Is this what dying feels like?*

I didn't feel like I was dying. Getting around was harder than it used to be, of course. I was awkward on the phone, stumbling over my words and struggling to find the right rhythm for my slowed, slurred speech. If I didn't pace myself carefully, I would be breathless by the end of the sentence.

But *dying*? No.

Surely, I would have felt a major shift in my body if I were dying, some signal that it was shutting down. But I felt like myself. A slower, clumsier, more frustrated version of myself, but myself, nonetheless. *I must be in denial. That's the first stage of grief, right?*

Most of the time, the thoughts in my head were a carousel of unproductive questions and mean thoughts:

Am I dying?

Probable ALS means you are probably dying.

I don't feel like I'm dying.

I don't look like the ALS patients I see online, with all their tubes and machines.

Yeah, but you walk with a cane, just like everyone else at PT. Plus, your speech sucks.

I can't believe I used to be an athlete.

Was that really only last year? You're so much weaker. Because you haven't been working out. Or—because you're dying.

I must be in denial.

God, I miss running.

I also spent quite a lot of time dissecting the phrase *probable ALS* in my mind, which always ended in a question mark—probable ALS? How long would I have to wait around to find out whether probable ALS was "real ALS" or "not ALS"? Did I have two to five more years to live or a normal lifetime with decades left? Probable ALS was disorienting.

∾

Adding to the disorientation, David and I had our first visit to the ALS Clinic: a one-stop shop for all things ALS.

As the nurse led us through the maze of walkways to a small exam room, she explained how the ALS Clinic worked. We would remain in the exam room while practitioners from PT, speech, occupational therapy, respiratory therapy, nutrition, and social work cycled through to talk to us.

"No need to move around or make separate appointments. We bring everything straight to you," the nurse said, smiling. Maximum efficiency, I liked it.

Clicking through my chart on her computer, she confirmed my name and birthdate, and then asked, "Do you have an advance directive?"

I looked at her blankly. "What's that?"

The nurse stopped clicking and looked up.

"Well, it's a legal document. It spells out your medical care wishes. It includes a living will, which specifies whether you want to be resuscitated, whether you want to be an organ donor—that kind of thing."

My blood ran cold. I had not even been fully diagnosed with ALS, and I was already supposed to know what to do with my body when I died?

"Um, I, um," I stammered.

David jumped in. "She's only been diagnosed with *probable* ALS."

Her brow furrowed slightly, then softened.

"I understand. We like to have our patients think about these issues early on so the documents are in place."

"I have a will from when I bought my first house," I said, trying to be helpful. *People-pleasing-checklist Andrea, right here.* My face reddened when I realized how ridiculous I sounded.

"That's a good start. You'll want to make sure that's up to date. You'll also want a power of attorney for someone to make medical decisions if you're unable to do so." She turned back to her computer screen, presumably to note that I didn't have those documents.

Great. I am already failing at dying.

The six appointments that followed were a blur. Three hours in that tiny room answering questions.

Each specialist opened with the same question: "How are you doing?" *What kind of a question is that? How do you think I'm doing?*

"I'm fine," I responded each time.

Then came a laundry list of topics to discuss: power wheelchairs, shower benches, house renovations, support groups for patients with ALS and their caregivers, and a computer screen I could control with my eyes to speak for me. The nutritionist mentioned buying a Vitamix—*hey, I always wanted one of those!*—to blend foods so I could suck them through a straw when I could no longer eat.

"You can even liquefy chili!" she said brightly. *Ugh, never mind about the Vitamix.*

Each specialist repeated this exact line: "The key to managing this disease is staying ahead of it."

Which led to some version of "I know it's early, but . . ." or "You don't need this yet, but . . ." followed by another way David and I should be preparing *now* for the imminent failure of my body. Then they ran through lists of practical adaptations or technological solutions to keep me moving, eating, communicating, and living in the house—the one we had just bought two months ago.

The practitioners all ended with "I know this is a lot of information to take in at once." *You think?*

David furiously scribbled notes throughout each appointment.* I pushed away thoughts like *You have the wrong room* and *This is not my life.* Hours in, I was unable to concentrate. I resorted to mostly one-word responses. My stomach grumbled. *Why didn't you eat lunch?* A migraine formed behind my right eye.

Even though I wanted out of that tiny room, we were committed to gathering as much information as possible.

Suddenly, a large woman exploded into the room and dismissed the nutritionist—mid-sentence—with a wave.

I would have jumped off the table if I hadn't been numb. Instead, I stared at her. *What have I done wrong now?*

"I'm just going to take over here and see if we can move things along," she said, plopping down at the computer. She introduced herself as the clinic director. Apparently, we were taking too long with the practitioners. We had caused the clinic schedule to fall behind.

"Let's see if we can get you out of here. What questions do you have for me?"

The only issue we had not discussed was the most important thing.

I took a deep breath, and said, "Well, before all this started, we were ready to try for a baby."

The director swiveled her chair from the computer to face me.

"What?" she blinked.

"Um, well . . . it's just that I've only been diagnosed with probable ALS. So if we're going to try to have a baby, it seems like now is the best time," I said, picturing the empty tabbed section at the end of my orange notebook. In my mind, it was already labeled *Baby*.

The director looked at me like I had sprouted another head right there in the exam room. Or sprouted a baby. Shock and horror.

---

* In hindsight, he didn't need to worry so much about capturing everything. We would listen to basically the same information, suggestions, and warnings about my imminent decline at each ALS Clinic visit every three months for years to come. *Talk about sucking the hope out of somebody.* If all you are told (by the *experts*) is how you are going to decline, how could there be any other outcome than to do so? I wish I could have had a physician or specialist at this phase really look at me, really hear me and David, and ask us what we were struggling with. Then they could have helped us by anticipating the *next* immediate step—not all of the steps at once. People living with ALS don't need an overwhelming list to go home with when they have an already overwhelming disease moving at a rapid pace.

When she spoke, her voice was lower and slower. "I don't think you understand."

From the looks David and I gave her, we obviously didn't understand at all. She continued. "You could be paralyzed by the time that baby comes."

I looked at David for help, my face crumpling in unexpected pain. He understood my glance. *What? Was motherhood already over for me?*

"But considering she hasn't been fully diagnosed with ALS, what sorts of things should we be thinking about if we were to move forward?" A practical question. *I love that David is a lawyer who interviews people for a living. Move forward. Yes. With a baby. Yes.*

"Well, you'd need lots and lots of help. Like round-the-clock care for both you"—she gestured to me—"*and* the baby. Because you (another gesture in my direction) might not be able to hold a baby or nurse one . . . or anything. You'd basically need a family member or two living with you."

God, no.

"And you'd definitely be a high-risk pregnancy, so let me see here . . ." she said, scrolling through her phone. Her voice resumed its normal, brisk speed. She was back in charge.

She gave us the name and number of an obstetrician specializing in high-risk births, saying, "I haven't talked to her in ages. She might be retired now for all I know."

The director confirmed from my file that I tested negative for the SOD-1 and C9orf72 genetic mutations associated with hereditary ALS.

"Researchers have found many, many more genes than those two, though. I think they're up to about thirty possible ones," she warned us.

We were out of questions. She ended the appointment.

⬤

After the events of the ALS Clinic, David and I carried a new, acute attentiveness in our marriage. Of how little time we might have left together. Neither of us wanted to waste it bickering about dishes and laundry.

We talked more. The "how was your day" question was no longer an automated response after work. Neither was a hug and kiss. We searched each other's faces for signs of cracking under the weight of our ordeal. We listened to each other express the litany of thoughts we could not say to anyone else.

"He was an asshole all day because he has to reschedule his vacation around this client meeting. I mean, I get it, but like seriously, get over yourself. You're still going to Cancun!" he said.

"Her posts drive me up the wall! Just stop whining about how hard it is to raise your children. Be grateful you have them and they're healthy!" I said.

The bond between us grew alongside our mutual distaste for everyone else's external griping. People just didn't understand how lucky they were to be alive and bored, with an entire future ahead of them.

David and I negotiated the practicalities of how life needed to change, but we did so without arguing. When David expressed concern about my climbing our front steps with no railing, I agreed to walk around to the back door, even though I considered it annoying and unnecessary. I agreed to prep dinner; he agreed to cook it. I had already stopped handling the cat litter in anticipation of my future pregnancy; he agreed to take over the smelly chore in perpetuity.

On weekends, we checked out new restaurants in downtown Silver Spring and explored the little farmers market. We bought furniture and decorations for our new house, since we had expanded from our cramped one-bedroom in Chinatown to four bedrooms on three floors. I was amazed at how smoothly our decision-making went. As newlyweds struggling to blend our lives and our stuff (only five years earlier), we argued over comforters and artwork for the walls. That stuff—literally just stuff—no longer mattered.

Our favorite weekends were spent with David's sister, her husband, and their two kids. Their two-bedroom townhouse in DC was tight quarters, so they loved coming to our sprawling suburban house with its big, fenced-in backyard. Our nephew and niece played freeze tag in the backyard for hours. When we all went inside, the quirky trilevel house (with its many closets) was perfect for hide-and-seek.

Mostly, the kids ran everywhere they could: inside, outside, around our huge finished basement with no furniture, screaming at the top of their lungs as their daddy and David chased them. My sister-in-law and I watched from a safe corner, laughing until our sides ached.

These weekends of laughter relieved my biggest fear.

I had been afraid David and I would never be able to duck out from under the looming shadow of ALS. I thought, *I'll never have another purely happy moment. From now on, the best I can feel is bittersweet.*

But the truth? The happy moments were purer and sweeter than ever before. That is, until Dad decided to change out the locks on our doors.

CHAPTER 10

LOCKS

Post–Probable ALS Diagnosis: July 2014

In an effort to restore our relationship with my parents, David and I invited Mom and Dad from North Carolina to our new house in Maryland.

I figured we could do what we *all* did best: work.

While David was at the office, Mom prepared a nice lunch for the three of us to eat outside on the patio. As we ate, we discussed what needed to be done. I made a list. My number one priority was to unpack the remaining boxes. This "simple" task was taking me forever with only one hand, since the other hand propelled the cane.

However, Mom-the-Realtor had a different number one for the list. Locks simply *must* be changed after purchasing a new house.

"You never know how many spare keys are floating around," she said. "Neighbors, cleaners, and dog walkers all have one. It's expensive, but your dad can do it. That'll save you a couple hundred bucks on a locksmith."

That seemed reasonable. *Okay, fine, locks moved to the top of the list.*

After lunch, Dad mowed the grass—one of his specialties. When he retired after teaching high school for forty years, he launched a business: Lawns by

Lytle. Tagline: *For a Yard You Can Enjoy.* After that, he was all over town with his push mower and a bandana tied around his neck. Inexplicably, he wore chef pants. The crazier the pants, the better: dancing jalapeños, tie-dye swirls, Day of the Dead skulls. I had to laugh. The man has style.

Mom and I unpacked boxes. Then Mom cooked dinner while I squeezed in a bit of work. We were all on our best behavior. Over dinner, we filled David in on the plans for the lock install the next morning.* An additional list for the hardware store was made. So far, so good. *Go team.*

After David left for work the next morning, Dad removed the doorknobs from three exterior doors and headed to the hardware store with Mom. After a long while, I looked at the clock. *Where are they?* They had left the house at 10 A.M. When they hadn't returned by 1 P.M., I texted Mom and learned they had been stuck in traffic for hours trying to reach the hardware store just a few miles away.

"We're coming back as quickly as we can—with lunch," she texted back.

When they still hadn't shown up by 4:30 P.M., I called David to vent. I also laughed a little, because this was classic Mom and Dad.

David, however, was not amused.

In fact, he was furious. He hung up with me, called Mom, and demanded they return home so she could accompany me to my acupuncture appointment while Dad put the new locks in before dark. They agreed to return home quickly.

Now is a good time to discuss David's obsession with locking doors.

He inherited the trait from his parents, who are similarly vigilant about their house alarm system, even though they live in an extremely safe, quiet neighborhood in an affluent suburb. David locks the car doors before putting on his seat belt and hits the door lock button a few more times while driving. Once he exits the car, he initiates an aggressive triple-lock sequence, clicking the key fob until the horn sounds (even though I have pointed out that one

---

* David disputes this alleged conversation. He claims he was not apprised of this plan. Which might explain what happened next.

button push is sufficient—no horn needed). He frequently gets out of bed after we turn out the lights just to check the front door, which is (of course) already locked. He doesn't have many compulsions like this, so I definitely tease him about it (as any good wife would do), which he takes in stride (as any good husband would do).

In contrast, my family has never cared about locks. When I was growing up, our back door was left unlocked for convenience. The garage door remained wide open. My parents only started closing the garage door after they found a deer nosing around inside.

I explained David's genetic door-locking disorder to Mom as we inched along in rush hour traffic on the way to acupuncture. Mom and Dad had shown up exactly ten minutes before I needed to leave. She politely relayed some of her conversation with David. I read between the lines to fill in the (not-so-polite) rest. She was tired and frustrated as well, but was clearly most surprised by David's anger.

Despite having a hot button, David doesn't get worked up about small stuff. The stakes must be high—or at least, high for him. When he is stressed out about something *big to him* that others don't think matters? Well, then he's likely to explode.

So to step inside dear, lock-obsessed David's psyche for a moment—imagine him leaving a house unlocked, because the locks had been *purposely* removed? Add in an eighty-hour-a-week stressful job and his wife's (probable) terminal illness—well, I think you understand.

From her relay of the call, I knew Mom absorbed David's outburst without fighting back. The same way she handled me when I got mad. She apologized and tried to explain (at which point I was certain David cut her off). For the first time, she must have questioned who her daughter had married, having never seen this side of him before.

This was weird. I wasn't the peacemaker; David was. He was the one to translate my fits of frustration to my bewildered parents. Andy and Sandy always wanted to do the right thing. And if whatever it was calmed their daughter down, it qualified as the right thing. David and I often wondered how my parents and I survived before he came into the picture.

After acupuncture, Mom and I returned home, and I reexplained David's lock obsession, this time to Dad. David—bless him—was still at the office.

Then I asked a simple question: "Why did a trip to the hardware store take all day?" *Literally.*

When Mom and Dad finally got to the store, the clerk informed them they could not replace the core in the doorknob (where the key goes in). The store could only duplicate keys. An employee knew someone who could do it for cheap, though: his instructor at the community college where he'd learned to cut keys. Which was how my parents ended up driving another forty-five minutes into Prince George's County trying to track down the professor of keymanship, or whatever his title was.

"Why didn't you just buy a whole new set of doorknobs? Wouldn't those have come with matching keys?" I asked. Neither had an answer for this. I sighed. *Work harder, not smarter. The family way. Seven hours later.*

Things were not going well for Dad, though. We found this out when Mom set the Chinese takeout on the table.

The doorknobs no longer fit in the holes. Yes, the same holes the same doorknobs left a mere twelve hours before. Dad's eyesight is pretty poor, so he had dragged over our torchiere lamps and put down a plastic tarp so the tiny screws he continued to drop wouldn't also roll away.

If my parents were surprised by my husband's anger that afternoon, they hadn't seen anything yet.

My David.

My dear, hardworking, lock-obsessed David arrived home at 9 P.M. After a long day at the office, a long commute on the Metro, and still facing a 10 P.M. conference call with clients in China . . . to find no locks on the doors.

His rage foamed out of his entire body. *A real live volcano. A volcano. I need to run. But I can't run. Oh my goddddd . . . here it comes . . .*

"I just do not see how this could have happened. We never *said* we needed new locks—*you* did. There is so much to do around here. Everything that doesn't get done, *I* have to do. *And now we have no locks on the doors!*" A vein popped out on his forehead. I swear I could see his heart pounding in his neck and in that vein.

"I'm just so, so sorry. I'm as sorry as I can be," Dad said quietly, so pathetically that my heart broke into a million pieces. "I never meant—"

"What are we supposed to do now?" David spat out, cutting him off.

"Well, I'm just so tired now, and I'm making mistakes. I think if I can start fresh in the morning, I can get it done."

"No," David said firmly. "We're hiring a professional locksmith. Which is what we should have done in the first place *if* we wanted the locks changed. Which we didn't."

"Okay, enough," I said, looking from Dad to David. "You said your piece. Go eat dinner and get ready for your call."

He glared at me. He assumed I would take his side and join in to yell at them. But I just couldn't. I wouldn't. I knew my parents tried as hard as they could. I knew they felt awful. Worse than that, it all felt like I was looking in the mirror. I could see clearly how *I* must have looked the countless times I had flipped out at them.

I cringed under the weight of my guilt.

Without another word, David stomped out of the room.

⁂

We woke the next morning to the sounds of my parents rustling in the kitchen.

David asked me to stay in bed so he could go out and apologize. He felt terrible, as I knew he would. So I rolled over and pretended to sleep as he left the room, then remained motionless and listened as hard as I could. I could not make out any of the words, but there was no yelling.

After twenty minutes or so, I couldn't stand it any longer. I propelled my cane into the kitchen. Mom and Dad's matching suitcases were sitting in front of the lockless front door.

"Everything okay?" I asked. Nodding and tense smiles all around.

"Uh, yeah. I think so," David said. "I'm going to get ready for work." An escape hatch.

"You guys okay?" I asked my parents when David left the room.

"I'm sure your dad could finish it," Mom said. "But David insists on paying a locksmith."

"Yeah, I know. He's as stubborn as I am sometimes," I said, attempting the tiniest of smiles. "But did he apologize?"

"Yes, he did," Dad said. "And so did we." But Mom's eyes didn't meet mine.

"Well, you guys don't need to leave right away, right? Maybe we could do some other stuff around here."

"We're not going to stay where we're not welcome," Mom said. A fact. The way she said it transported me straight back to the hotel interrogation room: "I accepted a long time ago that we weren't close." I put my hand on the kitchen table to steady myself.

"You're welcome to stay. I *want* you to stay," I pleaded. "I'm sorry this all happened." *I am sorry. I am always sorry.*

"We know you didn't mean for it to happen," Dad said. Mom said nothing.

I did not know how to make things better. But I felt the sand of our family dynamic shift treacherously beneath my already unsteady feet. I convinced them to at least stay for breakfast. While they pulled food out of the fridge and set the table, I checked on David.

❧

"She looked straight through me," David said, buttoning his shirt. "I apologized for blowing up at them. She said 'okay' and that was it. That was *it*. I mean, what more can I say?"

"I don't know. Maybe she just needs time to get over it. Just don't say anything to make it worse."

David shot me a look. "I shouldn't even be the one apologizing." A fact. Ugh. I hated this peacemaker shit.

After breakfast, everyone participated in a stiff, civil round of goodbyes at the front door. David apologized again, hugged each of my parents, and said he loved them. Dad hugged back and said he was sorry too. Mom went through the motions of a hug, then visibly recoiled inside of it. David's face took on a well-if-that's-how-you're-going-to-be expression. I stood in the middle of it all, just willing it to end.

David left quickly, opening the door by pushing the hole where a doorknob should have been.

CHAPTER 11

THE DIAGNOSIS (PROBABLY)

Diagnosis: August 2014

The door lock debacle hardened into a stalemate with my parents. David hadn't spoken to them in a month. I was a terrible peacemaker. But I was awesome at feeling guilty.

I communicated with my mother on my own, but it wasn't going well, either. She did not like the information I relayed about the ALS Clinic visit. She continued to prod me to get a second opinion from a different neurologist.

"That wishy-washy probable ALS diagnosis sounds like a cop-out," she said.

Although I agreed with her, the more she pressed, the more annoyed I got. If I really had ALS, and therefore two to five years to live, the last thing I wanted to do was spend my time going to different doctors, begging for a different diagnosis, and arguing with my mother. *I will probably drop dead in a doctor's office waiting room.*

Around this time, a trend started on social media: videos of people dumping ice water on their heads and talking about ALS. Two young guys with ALS, Pete Frates and Pat Quinn, launched the Ice Bucket Challenge to raise awareness and money for ALS research. They challenged their friends to post a video pouring ice water on their heads in twenty-four hours or pay $100 to an ALS charity. As a reward, the friends could issue the challenge to three new people of their choice. Most people received the ice dumping *and* donated to the cause—a pretty genius way to raise money.

Within weeks, the challenge went viral. Justin Timberlake challenged Jimmy Fallon and the Roots. Mark Zuckerberg challenged Bill Gates, who rigged scaffolding and a pulley system for his turn. Fire departments, sports teams, politicians, and thousands of ordinary people, all over the world, all repeating those three letters I had been obsessing over for months now.

A-L-S. For most people, the Ice Bucket Challenge was a silly game for a disease they had never heard of.

I'd never heard of ALS either. Until I found out it would (probably) kill me.

I watched every video I could find, focusing on the people with ALS. I stared at their wheelchairs, winced at the holes in their necks with tubes sticking out. I studied their slow, slurred voices to see if I recognized my speech patterns. I blinked, mirroring those individuals staring at computer screens where they spelled words with their eyes, no longer able to speak. *No way. This is not happening to me.*

I watched and rewatched photographer Anthony Carbajal's video.[1] It started out in the typical lighthearted fashion as he sported a pink bikini with "Kiss My ALS" on the back of his booty shorts.

Then the video took an awful, serious turn.

"I've been terrified of ALS my whole life," he said. He paused as his face crumpled into tears. "ALS runs in my family. My grandmother had it. My mom was diagnosed when I was in high school, and five months ago, I was diagnosed with it at twenty-six years old. ALS is so, so, so fucking scary, you have no idea." The video cut to Anthony at his mom's bedside. She was a rag doll; he picked up and moved her limp body to a chair so he could feed her through a tube connected to her stomach. *No way. This is not happening to me.*

The Ice Bucket Challenge went on to generate more than $220 million worldwide—about $110 million in the US alone. A staggering, game-changing amount, yet I knew, from my reading, that the pace of research was entirely too slow to save my life if I actually had ALS.

Seventy-five years had passed since Lou Gehrig's famous speech, where the longtime Yankees first baseman humbly said, despite his diagnosis: "Today I consider myself the luckiest man on the face of the earth."[2] I wondered what he would say if he knew there was still no effective treatment seventy-five years later.

The Ice Bucket Challenge made me a mini-celebrity among my friends. I was the only person they knew who may (or may not) have ALS. A few more friends poured ice water on their heads and dedicated the experience to me, which made me smile and feel a rush of love, but also made me feel like a fraud.

What if I don't have ALS? I thought, immediately followed by a scarier thought: *What if I do?*

⸺

As if my mama drama and mounting stress weren't enough, I started to receive mixed signals from the ALS Clinic.

Bonnie, my physical therapist, said at the end of one session, "I think we should get you into speech therapy."

"Why?"

"I'm noticing you're running out of breath when you speak. Also, your words are just a bit more slurred," she said. She offered to call the ALS Clinic and facilitate the process of getting me into speech therapy. As much as I hated to admit it, she was right, and I agreed.

A week later, I asked Bonnie about the status. Her brow furrowed.

"I thought you had said you hadn't been diagnosed with ALS," she said. *Right, probable ALS. But probably, ALS. Yes. No. Yes. No.*

I blinked at her.

Bonnie continued. "The clinic director said they don't recommend speech therapy for people with ALS. Instead, they steer patients toward phone apps that speak what you type, eye-gaze technology, things like that—none of which you need right now," she added quickly. I almost rolled my eyes. *Where have I heard that before?*

"But I only have probable ALS," I protested. I inwardly shuddered at the videos I had watched. The wheelchairs and the robot computer voices reading out what the person with ALS wanted to say.

"I think you need to talk to the neurologist again," she said. She tried to keep her face neutral, but the way she pursed her lips frightened me.

I replayed the conversation with Dr. Caustik from the last visit in my head. *Did she tell me I had ALS and I missed it? The most important news of my life? Is that even possible?*

I called my mother-in-law on the way home. I insisted we retrace what we both remembered from that conversation with Dr. Caustik in her office after the EMG test.

I said, "I asked her if it was ALS, right? And she said, 'What's the point of a diagnosis?' and then started talking about the ALS Clinic, right?"

"That's how I remember it," my mother-in-law said.

"And then Dr. Dave and David came back. And Dr. Caustik repeated her conclusion of probable ALS, right?" She agreed. *Okay, great.*

Then I got really angry.

How could four people with advanced degrees—one with a medical degree, mind you—have misunderstood Dr. Caustik? David and I called it probable ALS to everyone at the ALS Clinic—and no one corrected us? What does the word *probable* mean, anyway?

This was too much. The jackhammering of the question *What if?* in my brain had gotten too loud for me to think about anything else.

I called Dr. Caustik.

"I'd like to schedule another EMG," I said. "Living in limbo about whether it's ALS, PLS, or something else is keeping me awake at night."

There was a longer-than-necessary pause on the line before she responded.

"We can do another EMG," she said slowly. "But I don't expect it to be much different since it's only been a couple of months. We could at least go over the results again."

Well, *that* sounded ominous.

⁓

We invited my parents to the follow-up appointment, so Mom could see the EMG for herself and ask all of her questions. My anxiety was so high that I was willing to endure the horrific trifecta of painful needles, ham radio noises, *and* the stalemate with my mother, all at once.

David and I were fully prepared this time. Like a protest chant, we were ready: *We will not be blindsided by ALS! We will ask direct questions! We will receive clear answers! We will eat lunch beforehand!*

So I had the captive audience of Mom, Dad, and David as Dr. Caustik stuck her vicious little needles into my muscles and told me to flex. The crackly, static ham radio noise resumed.

This go-around, I understood what the static noises meant. I knew that the needle inside the flexed muscle would make noise. Then when I relaxed, the sound *should* quiet down after a beat. A healthy muscle is "quiet" after it relaxes. An unhealthy, potentially ALS-indicative muscle would continue to make noise after it relaxed.

I tried to leave my body, but with each stab, I felt mildly vindicated. Maybe now Mom would understand why I did not want to spend the rest of my life going to new doctors.

I sat in the pain. I sat in the noise that I begged to stop. The crackling that continued where a void of silence should be. There was definitely more noise than the first EMG. *More noise.* Not good.

For the benefit of the newbies in the room, Dr. Caustik explained the test as she went along, poking me and talking over the noise of the crackling static. With the course of my life hanging in the balance, the drawn-out excruciating truth was coming at a rate that was simultaneously too fast, too slow, and all the speeds in between.

She showed my family the real-time results on her screen.

The indications of ALS in my arms and legs.

But no indications of ALS in my back or my stomach.

"One region of the body, that's possible ALS," Dr. Caustik said. "We've got two regions, so that's probable ALS. To get to a definitive diagnosis of ALS, you need three regions in the body. But I'm guessing you don't want me sticking needles in your tongue."

Seriously? I almost exploded at her. The concept that had tortured me for months seemed so simple now. Probable rain didn't mean a chance of no rain. Probable just meant it hadn't rained *yet.*

I was ready to ask the critical question. To know the truth.

Looking her straight in the eyes, I asked, "Do I have ALS?"

"Yes," she said simply.

Reporters often ask how I felt at *that* moment—the moment I was diagnosed with ALS.

That moment doesn't exist for me. That moment is sand slipping through my fingers.

That moment is the long, twenty-month journey leading up to it. An animated flip-book of moments revealing the entire story: a stuck finger in the pool, tight hamstrings and balance issues during a half-distance triathlon race, a fall in the middle of the street, a spinal tap, appointments with five different neurologists, mind-numbing fear, the locks, my parents, scene after scene of confusion and terror.

That moment doesn't matter, except to underscore this one singular thought that pushed out all others: *I have no more time to waste in this life.* I had wasted the summer worrying, and the news came anyway.

Mostly, I tell reporters, I remember walking out of the appointment into the warmth of the August sunshine, talking to my parents and husband, and eating pizza that night. Walking, talking, eating. Who knew how much longer I would be able to do any of those things?

There was no fighting that night. The stalemate had been abandoned. I had my people, and they had me.

So actually, *that* was the moment I realized that, for all ALS destroys, it can't take away my family or the sun warming my face. As long as I live.

"How did you feel the day *after* your diagnosis?"

This is the far more interesting question reporters never ask. Not the moment you learn you're going to die, but the first day you wake up with that knowledge and have to figure out how to go on living.

I stretched out in the unfamiliar white sheets of our hotel bed, blinking my eyes, unsure of what to do next. Unsure of how to feel. The paralyzing anxiety of not knowing was gone. The what-if questions bouncing off the walls of my brain for almost a year had quieted at last. I assumed a soul-crushing depression would now descend. So I waited.

David felt me stirring and rolled over. He pulled me close and kissed my temple. His familiar, home-like, intoxicating smell drew me in, and I snuggled against his chest.

"What do you want to do today?" he asked softly.

I had no idea. My calendar ended yesterday. What do you do the day after you're told you're going to die?

We had both taken the day off work. I could not remember the last time we had a full day all to ourselves with absolutely no plans.

I could tell just by the sun streaming through the curtains that it would be a hot one. A sultry end-of-summer day, the kind that when you were a kid you knew meant summer would be ending soon and you never wanted to let go of. When you started pining for one last adventure before school starts.

"I want to go to a water park," I said.

"What?" David started laughing.

We didn't go to a water park. We did grown-up, responsible things like calling the insurance company and filling my prescription for Riluzole, the only FDA-approved drug at the time for ALS. Riluzole extends the life expectancy for people with ALS by two to three months, which shocked me when Dr. Caustik first mentioned it. I figured the next word after "two to three" was going to be "years," not "months." Why even bother tacking on another couple of months of suffering to a paralyzed, helpless existence? What good does that do?

But David's question stayed with me, knocking around inside my head. *What do you want to do today? What do you want to do today?*

It might as well have been, *What do you want to do with the rest of your life?* Since apparently there weren't too many todays left for me.

I want to do another triathlon, came the answer from deep in my soul.

⁂

Six months earlier, I had texted my friend Julie: "I have a crazy idea. Let's do a triathlon!"

At the time, I was feeling optimistic. Back when I thought I had overly tight hamstrings and some weird athletic injury going on. Back when I was just a medical mystery, before the criminal misnomer of probable ALS took over my brain.

After some prodding, Julie had said yes to her first triathlon. Which I knew she would—she is that kind of friend. Also, I am pretty good at talking people into things.

We picked the women-only Ramblin' Rose triathlon in Chapel Hill, North Carolina—which was scheduled for October. As a super-sprint tri (250-yard pool swim, 9-mile bike, and 2-mile run), it's a great beginner triathlon, a doable challenge for moms with kids, and a fun alternative to the stressful race environment for experienced triathletes.

But as spring turned into summer, aside from my half-hearted swimming routine, I wasn't really training; my doctors had told me not to.

The goal of finishing another triathlon faded with my muscle strength, overshadowed by probable ALS and an unknown future.

Until I discovered a man named Jon Blais and his connection to number 179.

Two Weeks before Diagnosis: August 2014

I began playing the French horn in fourth grade. In seventh grade, my frugal-yet-ever-supportive parents bought me a brand-new Holton Farkas French horn, model *179*. That year, I came in second in the all-state band competition. My score: *179* out of 200. Since that time, 179 has been my lucky number. Such a middle school thing to do. Weird, sure, but I believed in this number 179. Like a friendly little wave from the universe, I saw it often—on license plates, house numbers, and price tags. I chose it whenever possible for race numbers, lotteries, and the like.

Two weeks before my follow-up appointment with Dr. Caustik, I had searched for "triathlon" and "ALS" on the internet. I thought maybe I could find a race that benefited an ALS charity . . . or one that would allow a disabled athlete—since that appeared to be where I was headed.

The Blazeman Foundation popped up in my search. Their website was scattered with photos of the number 179, on race bibs. An embedded video of someone on a bike with the number.

My body flooded with goosebumps.

This is how I first learned about Jon Blais, also known as "the Blazeman." Jon Blais became an IRONMAN in 2005—finishing the race of 2.4-mile swim,

112-mile bike, and 26.2-mile marathon at the World Championship in Hawaii—five months after being diagnosed with ALS at the age of thirty-three. *My age.*

I scarcely breathed watching the entire six-minute compilation video of Jon's story broadcast during NBC Sports coverage of the IRONMAN World Championship. I sat transfixed, my hand covering my mouth.

"Competitor 179, Jon Blais," commentator Al Trautwig said, as the scene opened with Jon on his bike. "Essentially, Jon has been given a death sentence . . . but Jon's fatalistic view is based on reality. . . . Which right now involves . . . realizing that—today—he can still do this. Because today is what he has. It's what we all have."

The lump rose in my throat, and my goosebumps returned.

As the next scene jumped forward to nightfall, Jon's voiceover read a poem he'd written. On screen, Jon jogged toward the finish line as the cheers grew louder:

> *Understand that this is not a dress rehearsal.*
> *That this is it . . . your life.*
> *Face your fears and live your dreams.*
> *Take it in.*
> *Yes, every chance you get.*
> *Come close,*
> *And, by all means, whatever you do*
> *Get it on film.*

A few steps in front of the finish, Jon knelt down on all fours and rolled across the finish line. He stayed on the ground, overcome with emotion and exhaustion, as his mother crouched down to place a lei around his neck.

"Jon Blais, *you are an IRONMAN!*" boomed the legendary announcer Mike Reilly.

Tears streamed down my face. Chills ran up and down my body as if I had gone into shock. Which really, I *had.*

Jon lived fewer than two years after his performance in Kona. Pro and amateur triathletes still perform the Blazeman Roll to this day, even though Jon had been dead for more than ten years. He remained the only person with

ALS to complete an IRONMAN unaided until 2017. The World Triathlon Corporation retired bib number 179, except when requested by an athlete racing for a charitable cause, usually ALS.

I had no idea of Jon's story—or ALS—when I had requested number 179 for my first Olympic-distance triathlon in 2013. My lasting memory of that race: apologizing to the race volunteers out on the course for being so darn slow. Embarrassed, I cried in the car all the way back to the interstate. *I had no idea.*

He knew he was going to die, but Jon chose how he would be *remembered.* I watched that video over and over. I memorized Jon's words and his poem, believing there was too much coincidence to ignore. I couldn't run, but I *could* learn Jon's courage.

I couldn't do an IRONMAN, but I *could* do a sprint triathlon to raise money for ALS research through the Blazeman Foundation—Jon's foundation.

At least a triathlon could be a happy memory for when I was stuck in a wheelchair, paralyzed. And something for David to remember when I was gone.

⤫

By the time I was diagnosed in August, the Ramblin' Rose triathlon was a mere five weeks away.

Swimming would be fine in the race. The run? Well, there would be no running, considering I walked with a four-footed-bariatric-behemoth of a cane. But I could still walk.

That left the bike, which was the most problematic. All I could offer a bike was shaking legs, trouble dismounting, and low-speed tip-overs. And I wasn't supposed to fall, remember?

With David spotting me, I attempted to get on my road bike using the indoor bike trainer—a type of bike stand that allows you to ride indoors.

But even a bike that didn't move was a no-go. My inner thighs were too tight to stretch over the top bar and my legs shook uncontrollably.

David and I looked at each other. *Well, shit.*

I rationalized that a heavier bike with wider tires would be more stable.

The next day, we drove out to an empty DC Metro parking lot so I could try what I considered to be the bariatric-behemoth-cane equivalent: the Capital Bikeshare bike.

A CaBi (rhymes with crabby), as it is affectionately known in DC, is a rental bike intended for short trips. Local governments created the program to keep additional cars off the road. CaBis feature three speeds, a heavy step-through frame, and wide tires.

I was apprehensive. David was more apprehensive. His apprehension ratcheted up mine. *Okay, well, let's see what happens.*

We started in the grass. David held the bike. I stepped through and clumsily climbed onto the seat. I put one foot on the pedal and tried to make it move while David held the back of the bike, like a father teaching his child to ride without training wheels.

I don't know whether it was him holding the bike, the CaBi's heaviness, the grass, our mutual anxiety, or ALS, but I could not get it to move. The bike and I wobbled for a moment and then toppled over into the grass.

We tried a couple more times, but each attempt was worse. My legs began shaking wildly, which added to the futility.

Finally, on the ground with tears in my eyes, I looked up at David. "I'm done."

Silently, we locked up the bike in the rental rack and walked back to the car.

As soon as we were in the car, I started wailing. Frustration, anger, and sadness exploded forth from the center of my being with a force I'd never felt before. The tears seemed to come from everywhere. Every pore in my body cried. All the stored emotion and anxiety from the past year, our future that has disappeared, and with it, my last attempt at a triathlon. *Gone. Just gone.*

So this is how it is going to be from now on. One loss after another.

Next, ALS would attack my ability to walk, then to speak. Then take away my ability to eat, then to move, and finally, to breathe. That is ALS. *This is really happening to me.*

I knew David was crying too, but I couldn't look at him. If I added his pain on top of mine in that moment, it would have destroyed me. My body might have just blown apart, right there in the car.

I cried until there was nothing left of me. The hyperventilating sobs slowed because I didn't have any energy to sustain them any longer. We held each other then, both of us whimpering and sniffling.

What do you want to do today? The words took on a whole new, woefully sad meaning.

CHAPTER 12

RIDING ON THREE WHEELS

September 2014

I told Julie the triathlon was off. As much as I wanted to do it—especially after learning about Jon Blais—I was unable to ride a bike of any sort. David and I had tried everything, including the CaBis. I told her that story too.

"What about something with three wheels—like a trike?" Julie asked.

"A what?" I pictured the big red tricycles we had ridden together around the preschool playground—thirty years ago when we first became friends.

"A trike. A three-wheeled bike," Julie said. "I found them online when I was trying to figure out what people with . . . um . . . mobility issues would use."

"Ugh," I said. "I don't know."

I promised to think about it.

Over the next few days, I realized this was my last chance to do another race, so what was holding me back? Pride? Ego? Feeling sorry for myself? I repeated the words that had come to me at the last visit with Dr. Caustik—*that* moment when I understood my ALS diagnosis: *I have no more time to waste in this life.*

Besides, while I hadn't been training, Julie had. For her first triathlon, she'd taken swim lessons and bought a bike. In order to best support me.

Finally, I couldn't let go of the connection to number 179 and Jon Blais. He had the courage to do a full IRONMAN with the world watching. He left a legacy of $2 million for ALS. I could make *my* journey mean something too.

I wrote a blog post that confirmed my ALS diagnosis and announced my attempt at one last triathlon to raise money for ALS research. A call to action for "Team Drea," referencing the T-shirts David had made to kick off the Year of the Triathlon. I stated that beyond spending quality time with family and friends, my priority now was to be of service. To make something positive out of my journey with ALS. I relayed Jon's story, his impact on me, and the significance of the number 179.

My friends and family leapt into action, donating money, and sharing my writing. People I hadn't talked to since high school donated. Strangers donated.

In two weeks, almost $10,000 poured into the online fundraiser. I felt a little surge of elation with each donation—humbling kindness, love, and support. Just when I needed it most.

✑

The next weekend, David and I purchased a recumbent trike.

Even the sticker-shock price tag of $2,300 wasn't a deterrent, because we were both so committed to the mission of the triathlon. *Hell, we can use my retirement savings,* I thought.

"Given your size, we'll start you in the Catrike Pocket," said the shop owner as he led us to the trikes. I stared down at the smallest of Catrike's fleet, a spritely neon green trike, also called a "tadpole" because of its two wheels in the front and one wheel in the rear. But with thirty speeds, time-trial bar-end shifters, and disc brakes, this was definitely not my tricycle from childhood.

My heart skipped a beat. *It is . . . adorable.*

After a quick briefing, I took a test drive around the parking lot. I picked it up quickly. Within minutes, I was flying around the parking lot doing loopy figure eights. Zooming mere inches from the asphalt was thrilling—like driving a go-cart. Or a sled. I beamed from ear to ear, unable to hide my glee.

I looked up to the clear sky and felt something familiar bubbling up inside of me: the freedom of motion. The sensation of slicing through slick-calm water in the bow of a crew shell. The meditation of swimming, submerged beneath the surface where the world was quiet, completely in charge of my own destiny.

I hadn't realized how much I had craved this independence. Not a patient, an athlete. Not scared, powerful. Not disabled, free to explore—as long as I put in the work to overcome whatever lay ahead of me.

David joined me on a David-sized trike. We were in a real-life game of Super Mario Kart, chasing each other all over the parking lot, laughing hysterically. The shop owner had the expression of a proud parent, looking at his two new converts to the sport of triking. When we rode beyond an appropriate test drive time, I reluctantly pulled up to the shop owner's feet—still grinning.

So, we committed to the little neon green trike. With a mix of amazement and horror, David and I watched the shop owner pull out a hacksaw and cut off the end of the boom connecting the pedals to make the trike even more "compact." Apparently, I was that short.

"Hey, less weight to carry," he joked. The thing was only twenty-nine pounds to start with.

With the trike loaded into our station wagon, we headed home. As I drove, I glanced through the rearview mirror at the trike. Then over at David, who had fallen asleep. I was so in love with them both.

CHAPTER 13

A FINISH LINE

October 2014

Julie and I entered the indoor pool area to start the Ramblin' Rose Triathlon.*

The swim was "snake" style. One at a time, a competitor swam down one length of the pool, ducked under the lane rope, and swam back—snaking across the pool from one side to the other.

When the swimmer made it halfway down the first lane, a race official shouted "Go!" to the next woman in line. The result? Splashing, flailing arms, and kicking legs everywhere.

As we waited, I watched women of all ages, colors, shapes, sizes, and abilities launch themselves into the pool, while women waiting in line cheered them on. *When else do you get to see something like this?* Mesmerized, I tried to take it all in for the very last time.

When I was told to go, I launched myself into the fray.

---

* And David, always my protector, who talked his way into the pool area even though spectators weren't allowed. He stood along the wall "just in case."

My body felt strangely disjointed. My breathing was shallow and all wrong. I swallowed, snorted, and coughed water. Fear gripped my muscles and wouldn't let go. I had to pause at the end of each lane to relieve the bottleneck of swimmers treading water behind me. Everyone was friendly, which helped me feel a tad less mortified. *So much for all my swim training.*

Sweet relief to be out of the pool and in the transition area. *My trike!* With not a cloud in the sky, the sun warmed my body and spirit as Julie and I set out.

I enjoyed every inch of those nine miles of asphalt streaking beneath my tires. So much had been taken away from me in the past year—I reveled in the feeling of getting it back, for even one day. Sitting in that hospital room five weeks ago, I never dreamed I would have this much fun again.

I didn't realize how far we were behind everyone else, until some bike escorts joined us and I glimpsed flashing blue lights in my rearview mirror. We were last—what every triathlete dreads.

It was such a blast that I really didn't care, except I hated inconveniencing the volunteers and staff waiting on me. *People pleaser, always.*

Finished with the bike-trike portion, we still had the "run" to do. By now, the other racers had finished—the swim, the bike, *and* the run. I was fighting my own legs while the other athletes were sitting at Sunday brunch, eating pancakes and sipping mimosas.

"Feel free to pack everything up. No need to wait on me to finish," I had told Amy, the race director, when we'd met her at packet pickup. "I'm sure I'll get there, I just don't have any idea how long it will take."

Off my trike, it was time to see what my walking legs could do.

Only two miles. I repeated to myself. *It's only two miles.*

Two trekking poles had replaced my trusty four-footed cane. They clanked and scraped on the concrete, providing little assistance. Because, apparently, my legs had decided they were done for the day. *Come on, legs.* I urged them along with my brain. All ten toes cramped in my shoes. Both feet dragged me forward slowly. My knees locked out with every step.

Yet, I knew I wouldn't quit.

It was crazy that only one year before I had finished a half-distance triathlon—and hadn't been last. My brain was difficult like that—remembering things so vividly, reminding me of how things used to be.

Stop it. I shut down the inner dialogue. I would not fight myself. That was not the point of this race.

All I had to do was put one foot in front of the other, over and over again. Julie and I moved like turtles, but we *were* moving.

Near the finish, several of Julie's friends joined us. Other race finishers tagged along, too. Race volunteers showed up, but it turns out, they thought we were lost. I was touched, and a little embarrassed. *Quite the entourage!* I tried to smile to let everyone know I was okay without having to talk. While Julie was used to my slurred speech, others were not.

Although I knew our friends and families would be waiting, I didn't expect anyone else to be at the finish line. But as we rounded the final block, I heard loud music. Spectators and triathletes (who hadn't gone to brunch, after all) were dancing in the parking lot. As we approached the finish line, the dancers parted, the music boomed, and the entire crowd cheered—some crying.

With Julie supporting me on one side and David on the other, I walked slowly through the pandemonium. "We Are the Champions" blasted at full volume. *I can't look around. I will lose it.*

As I crossed the finish line, David lifted me off the ground in a bear hug. Mom and Dad shoved flowers into my arms, my mom hugging me even harder than David. Construction paper confetti rained down on us. It took me a moment to recognize it was the same construction paper confetti Julie and I had cut up at our New Year's Eve sleepovers—in *middle school.* Julie's mom had saved it all these years and brought a bag for the occasion. Later at lunch, someone anonymously picked up the tab for our entire table of eight.

That finish line forever changed me. I felt something reverberate through my whole body and soul. The support, energy, and love coming from every direction, every person, everywhere I looked—it was the very best of humanity. Compassion. Power. *Life.*

All that goodness directed straight at me.

The spark ignited. The crowd around me proved I could inspire people with my story; my friends and family proved I could raise money for ALS research. I was officially illuminated from the inside out.

Pride and humility made room for each other, united by an overwhelming sense of love from my grateful, still-beating heart. I felt so much love. Love for my sport, family and friends, fellow competitors, everyone who donated,

Jon. I felt so much love for David and his support as we bought that little green trike. I felt love for all the spectators who stayed to give a dying woman and her family a beautiful, happy memory to last a lifetime—no matter how long or short that would be.

⁂

When all the congratulatory messages, praise, and photos appeared on social media, I struggled to find the right words to describe the experience.

"It was the most extraordinary day of my life" is where I settled. *The most extraordinary experience I never even saw coming.*

As the commotion and elation from finishing the race quieted down, I searched for meaning in all that had happened—from ALS to Jon to that finish line spark.

"Is this a self-fulfilling prophecy? Is this God's plan? Have I been appointed this job? I think about that a lot," Jon had said in the NBC video.

The cosmic connection with Jon and the number 179 certainly set events in motion, but *I* was the one who had chosen to follow through with the trike and the triathlon. I could have shrugged off the coincidence, but I had chosen to give it meaning. The people cheering us at the finish line didn't know anything about the backstory of Jon or 179. What happened at the race was beautifully, extraordinarily spontaneous.

It felt new and different, like a springboard—but a springboard to what, exactly?

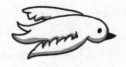

CHAPTER 14

FALLING

November 2014

In the Hallmark movie version of my story, that finish line would have changed everything:

> WOMAN WITH ALS FINISHES TRIATHLON, REALIZES SHE'S
> AN INSPIRATION, WAKES UP EACH DAY READY TO FACE HER
> FUTURE WITH COURAGE! THE STRAINS IN HER RELATIONSHIPS
> WITH HER PARENTS ARE INSTANTLY REPAIRED! SHE HAS LET
> GO OF GUILT AND FEAR AND SELF-PITY ONCE AND FOR ALL!
> SHE LIVES OUT HER DAYS WITH GRATITUDE AND PURPOSE!

But this is a real and true story, not a Hallmark movie.

And as magical of an experience as the triathlon had been, it could only buoy our spirits for so long. Nothing about our day-to-day reality had, in fact, changed. I was still on schedule to die in two to five years.

Work was becoming a nightmare.

My voice was getting worse. I concentrated on each syllable to avoid slurring the word. But when I focused too much on each syllable, I forgot to take extra pauses to breathe. So then, I ran out of air by the end of the sentence. And when I focused too much on how I sounded, I forgot what I was trying to say in the first place. Not a successful way to run a meeting.

My typing had slowed, too. I would draft an email response to a question, only to realize that by the time I finished, five follow-up emails had flown back and forth, rendering my email useless.

At this point, I was second-in-command for a small nonprofit that built a massive rating system to help cities measure their sustainability.* Our little team of five worked remotely across three time zones, so conference calls and emails were essential. The pace of our work increased with the publication of our rating system. We fielded questions, problems, complaints. There was a reason no one had created a municipal rating system this complex before.

When things got hard, my default solution had always been to work *harder*, put in longer hours. But the medication I took to relax my stiff muscles made me drowsy. When I took the pills later in the day so I could work longer, I couldn't speak clearly because my tongue and throat muscles remained locked down, tight.

My coworkers had been supportive throughout the past year, silently absorbing extra work as I disappeared to doctors' appointments, medical testing, and PT twice a week that took half the day. I knew my vanishing act was hard on them, but I was also incredibly frustrated. For all the work I had put into getting the project off the ground, I couldn't effectively supervise, communicate, or problem-solve like I used to.

I couldn't keep up. I couldn't even stay upright.

⚬⚬⚬

On a cold, gray day in December, I pushed my walker through the accessible automatic door into the massive lobby of the DC building. Our local employees met up every couple of weeks in a shared office space downtown. I was glad to be out and about—aiming to prove I could still contribute.

---

* Now called LEED for Cities.

The walker was new, as I had become too unstable to navigate the world with a cane. I loved my new walker, believe it or not. It was a relief to have more sure, stable footing.

Or so I thought.

I failed to lift the walker's back leg over the tiny lip of the entry mat. It caught underneath the mat, and I went sprawling.

Even on the way down, I looked up to see if anyone was watching.

Like most DC office buildings, the grand lobby's purpose was just to impress visitors. Thankfully, today there were none. I thought I was in the clear until the security guard, a small, middle-aged woman, came rushing over from behind her gatekeeping station by the elevators.

"I'm fine, I'm fine," I said before she reached me, waving her off. She would have none of it. Before I could register what was happening, she was behind me, hauling me upward by my armpits with surprising strength.

"We're going to need to do some paperwork on this one, yes, we will. You sure you're okay? I'll get the form. You need me to call someone? What floor you going to, honey? You wait right here. I'll get the paperwork."

"I'm fine, I'm fine," I protested, louder this time.

The security guard ran back to her guard post, and I chased her with my walker as fast as I could, talking to her back. The surge of adrenaline from the fall, combined with the alarm that my embarrassment was about to be recorded in print, made my speech even more pitched and breathy. But she wasn't listening to me anyway.

It took a full ten minutes of half insisting, half pleading, pen-in-hand but not going anywhere near the incident report form she shoved at me, to convince her that we did not need to report it. *Nope, no scrapes, I don't need a Band-Aid. Nope, you don't need to call anyone. I'm fine, I promise. Yep, yep, nope.*

I thought I was in the clear—again. I went upstairs and met my coworkers for the day.

Later, when our group walked out for lunch, I saw the security guard. She was checking credentials for some visitors, so I was sure I could fly under the radar. Just in case, though, I thrust myself into chatter with my coworkers. *If we can just make it past the security desk, then I will—*

"How you feeling, honey? You all right?" she asked me, killing the conversation as my coworkers looked at me curiously for an explanation.

"Yes, yes, I'm fine," I said, still walking, eyes fixed ahead. I would have waved her off if that didn't mean stopping the walker, risking further conversation.

So, I had to tell everyone the story at lunch. I tried to laugh it off, minimize it, blame it on the overzealous security guard. But I caught the look on my boss's face. She was concerned.

And that's the story of how I never went into that office again.

◈

I sat in our driveway for a long time when I arrived home. I was out of tears. I had cried all the way home in rush hour traffic.

As a cold, dark silence filled the car, I thought back to when I received confirmation of my ALS diagnosis. Why hadn't I fallen apart then? I had a track record of melting down over high school chemistry homework, wedding preparation drama, and all aspects of triathlon. And I had just spent an hour crying about an embarrassing fall. "Calm Under Pressure" was not my middle name. So.

Why was I calm when told I was going to die?

My most vivid memory of the diagnosis day was walking out of the hospital and feeling the warm sun on my face. I was grateful in that moment *for* that moment.

But why had I been so calm? The question rang in my ears.

Answer: I was accustomed to pushing against that emotional floor of self-pity, using a freak-out to bounce upward, to work harder to achieve whatever I wanted.

Answer: I spent nearly a year freaking out and pushing hard to get answers, to get a diagnosis. But there would be no bounce from the diagnosis. ALS meant death.

Softly, I exhaled into the darkness. Slipping on a rug would be a quaint problem in a couple of years—or months. When I couldn't use the bathroom on my own or feed myself. I did not have the luxury of self-pity anymore. I could not implode after each humiliating incident that lay ahead.

I heard the cold truth in my own head. There would be no bounce. It would only get worse. My fate was sealed, and so was David's. He would be under so much stress in the coming years as our only source of income, responsible for running the house on his own, being my primary caregiver, worrying about me, burying me, picking up the pieces of his life after I died, and figuring out how to go on. And I couldn't do anything about any of it.

I paused in the dark and felt a small shift. I exhaled again. A breath of knowing.

New answer: I could control my attitude. I could control the freak-outs. If I could be happy—or at least not fall apart over every new incident—that would be one less thing for David to worry about. If I could create happy memories for us, like the triathlon and joy of playing with our new kitten, maybe that would ease the burden I would become. *Already am.*

We could be depressed, or we could enjoy the time I had left.

The time would pass either way.

CHAPTER 15

WHERE THERE'S
A WILL

December 2014

My Christmas gift to David was a flash drive.

An hour-long slideshow movie set to our favorite songs with all 651 photos from our past twelve years together. If I was dead by next Christmas, at least he would have a record of our life together, organized in folders by month and year. (Of course it was organized.)

In David's childhood home, in the room with the Christmas tree, our entire family—both David's and mine—watched it together. We all cried.

If I ruined Christmas by screening this little movie, I refused to feel guilty about it. Everyone needed to feel the pain, to see my life slipping away. I needed everyone to reach the same point of acceptance that I felt sitting in the driveway after my fall in the office.

Acceptance with a capital *A*. *Acceptance.* This was happening. I was going to die.

The Acceptance would be painful for them. I knew and understood that. But I also knew it came with a silver lining I had discovered while putting together the slideshow: *it has been a beautiful life.* No matter what lies ahead.

ℂ

Around this time, I began to examine the language of social media posts in the ALS groups. Posts consistently used words like *horrific, terrible, tragic, devastating, heartbreaking, awful,* and *cruel* to describe ALS.

All absolutely accurate words, by the way. Accurate in ways I would no doubt learn in the coming months and years. Everyone is entitled to their experience, their feelings, and their personal translation of pain and grief.

Besides, I understood. Hope was the first thing to disappear when I was diagnosed. After all, with a 100 percent fatal disease, what was the point of Hope? Hope was a waste of time. Hope just cracked my heart into a million pieces. Hope would continue to break me over and over again as I continued to lose function and independence.

No Hope for me. I needed to be realistic. Pragmatic.

I needed Acceptance.

In this fragile time of Acceptance, I could *not* internalize all those negative words and emotions I read online. ALS impacted every single move I made during the day, so basically, ALS impacted my thoughts all day long. I could not let depressing words color every single move and thought for—*literally*— the rest of my life. I could not—would not—let that be the narrative inside my head.

I filtered my social media content. I blocked people. I joined some groups and left others. I let in information about the disease. I quietly scrolled past emotional posts from others.

And then, like a permission slip I didn't know I needed, I heard a radio interview. About a man who *voluntarily* stopped talking for seventeen years.

After witnessing an oil spill in San Francisco Bay in 1971, John Francis gave up motorized transport. For twenty-two years, he walked everywhere. Nicknamed the Planetwalker, he found himself speaking defensively about his choices, listening just long enough to know what he thought the other person was going to say, then tuning out to focus on his rebuttal. So John Francis stopped talking—for seventeen years.

Let me get this straight. All this time I've been worrying about losing my voice and this guy chooses *not to talk?*

Since I was on the way to losing my voice anyway, I tried to adopt some of his wisdom: listening to others, nature, myself, and also silence. I aimed to become more discerning with my words—whether spoken or written or eye-gazed or gestured or said to myself in my own head.

What I chose to think, what I chose to read, what I chose to say—if I was present and paid attention to these things, I could see that I had choices. *Choices*. Despite the death sentence of ALS.

While I could not control how or when ALS killed me, I could control how I approached every single day before it did.

I could not change the glacial pace of ALS research, but I could use my personal experience and fight to raise money to cure it.

I could not change that new people would be diagnosed every day, but maybe I could be a role model to whoever looked in my direction.

Then and there, I celebrated the beauty of choice, no matter how small.

⚬

With my renewed spirit of choices, I updated my will and finalized medical directives. Technically, I had a will. But the document from ten years ago that bequeathed my postage-stamp-sized, single-gal house and all worldly IKEA assets to my parents did not include David as my husband.

Gone was the cool, confident signature by that healthy Andrea person with her whole life ahead of her. Now that I knew for sure I would die—*soon*—I needed to get serious. In enough time to sign my own name.

Obviously, I had no medical directives in place—as established from the very first question at my very first ALS Clinic visit. (Okay, maybe it was the second question, after the inane "How are you doing?")

With a deep sigh, I opened the document the paralegal had sent. Glowing white-hot inside my brain were the questions from the ALS Clinic: *Who is my healthcare power of attorney? Do I want a Do Not Resuscitate (DNR) order? What do I want done with my dead body?*

At least I had a guide this time. It was time to become an A student at dying.

I breezed through the first part of the eleven-page questionnaire related to children and past marriages. Then I made a game of hunting down information and gleefully crossing through sections that didn't apply to me.

Eventually, the only remaining questions were about death itself—and the horrible process leading up to it. *Not just hypothetical death. My death. Soon.*

At least the route to my death was clear. I was not likely to be wheeled into the ER after a car accident with a life-threatening injury requiring heroic measures to keep my heart beating. A mental disability was also a very remote possibility—frontotemporal dementia (FTD) occasionally shows up in ALS, but not typically.

With ALS, my lungs would weaken until I could no longer survive without artificial means to breathe for me. I would likely already have a feeding tube so I wouldn't suffer from starvation or dehydration.

But what about a tracheostomy? A "trach" is a hole in the neck with a tube attached to a ventilator machine to breathe for the patient. Since the diaphragm and lungs weaken over time in ALS, at some point, this trach decision would be necessary.

After trach surgery, I would no longer be able to speak. Food, liquids, and medicine would be delivered through a feeding tube in my stomach. I would require around-the-clock care to monitor the machine and suction mucus so I wouldn't choke to death.

Only a very small percentage of ALS patients (around 10 percent) in the US opt for a trach. The other 90 percent don't want to die; they just can't afford to live. The cost of skilled nursing care (which isn't covered by insurance) can top $20,000 a month. In other countries, where this cost is covered by a national healthcare system, the percentage of ALS patients with trachs is higher.

But with a trach and a feeding tube, I would be alive. *Alive.* I would be able to think and communicate by typing with my eyes on a screen.

Could I really choose death instead of a trach? But what kind of life could I have, entirely imprisoned in my own body and fully dependent on machines and caregivers? I would be like a brain trapped in a body cast. Or would the choice come down to money? Lack of money seemed to be a ridiculous reason to die—but from the posts I'd read in online ALS groups, I knew many families faced that decision. Even if we could arguably afford it, could I live with the guilt of being such a financial burden?

I went back and forth in my head and just couldn't decide—certainly not permanently, in writing, at that moment. Thankfully, the attorney had told me it was okay not to know all the answers yet.

"The important thing is continuously communicating to your loved ones," he said. "As long as they know what you want, they can carry out your wishes. That's the point of the directive—so they can direct the medical staff on your behalf."

The only thing that remained on the forms was a final set of checkboxes. "Is your body to be buried or cremated?"

Oof. Another one I wasn't ready to answer.

Mom made her decision to be buried on a little island where their beach house is—she says that's where her spirit feels free. Dad chose cremation so he wouldn't take up any more room on Earth than necessary—really, I figured he wanted burial at sea to honor his Coast Guard and sailing days. Regardless, the fact that Andy and Sandy and their fifty-plus-year marriage would not be side-by-side for all of eternity released me from any romantic notions.

Besides, I wanted David to marry again after I was gone. What was the alternative—for him to carry on, lonely and miserable? *No.* I loved him enough that I wanted him to remarry, to finally experience having children of his own, and to live a long and happy life. But that made choosing my final resting place problematic—I didn't want him to be torn about where to be buried himself someday.

On the other hand, I hated the idea of having my ashes scattered. There would be nothing of me left. Like I never even existed.

I can't do this, I thought as the tears in the back of my throat threatened to choke me. *It's all too much. I'm only 33!*

I slammed my laptop closed, before I got sucked down into the pointless vortex of *why me?*

"Pace yourself," I said aloud, as if I was racing. There was only so much Acceptance I could handle at once.

I had choices—that was the important thing to remember.

As the saying goes: this would be a marathon, not a sprint.

❧

Having settled how I was going to die, I was ready to get on with living. David and I took a vacation to Turks and Caicos. Not up for a big, crowded resort, we opted for a rental house on the island of Grand Turk, the nation's capital, which appeared much less touristy than Providenciales.

Upon arrival, we immediately changed into our swimsuits, grabbed snorkeling gear, and headed out the back door to the Caribbean. I hung onto David's arm, which was part romantic gesture, part necessity. I couldn't stay upright on the shifting sand.

I'd imagined this moment for weeks. Before the trip, I had scrolled through tons of photos online of palm trees framing pristine white sand beaches that stretched into perfectly calm, clear blue water.

The landscape before our eyes was not at all the blissful tropical paradise I'd pictured. The overcast sky and the wind kicked up waves. Too choppy for snorkeling. We headed to the water for a dip, arm in arm.

It was only up to my knees when the undertow pulled me off-balance. *Whoosh.* I went down fast, then under the water. My back bumped and scraped along the sand, as my brain quickly flickered through visions of drowning and sea urchin impalement.

David yanked me up. I came out sputtering and spitting saltwater. I thought he was going to help me stand, but he picked me up and carried me to shore.

"What happened?" he asked, setting me down in the sand.

I was still coughing up water. I couldn't speak. We looked at each other, silently acknowledging how weak I had become. Ocean swimming (and knee-deep wading, apparently) were henceforth off the vacation agenda.

David moved away, ostensibly to collect our belongings, but I could tell he needed a minute to take in the enormity of what had just happened. I sat on the sand and stared at the waves. I shook my head, stunned at the speed at which my dream Caribbean vacation had imploded. I have deeply loved swimming in the ocean since childhood. The fact that my ocean days were over—forever—was just too much to take in. I needed a minute, too.

❧

Later that night, I awoke to the sounds of crashing waves outside our open window. I listened for a long while, soothed into pure stillness. So achingly peaceful. I was ready to doze again.

Except that I had to pee.

After hoisting myself out of bed, I rolled the walker toward the tiny bathroom. I had to leave the walker outside the threshold—it was too big to fit through the doorway.

Reaching for the sink, I misjudged the distance. I spun around on my way down, bashing the back of my head on the toilet paper dispenser. David came running in, breathing hard and full of adrenaline from being ripped awake.

"Are you okay? What did you hit?" he panted, flicking on the light and kneeling down.

With the wind knocked out of me, I gestured to the back of my head. He felt around my hair for a lump. When he pulled his hand away, it was streaked with blood. The color drained from his face.

"Shit! Oh my God. We've got to get you to the . . . hospital." He landed on the last word realizing there was certainly no hospital on this island. We also had no idea how to call for help. Would 911 work on Grand Turk?

"I'm fine, I'm fine," I said, but David wasn't buying it. He saw blood, after all.

He jumped up and ran out of the room, presumably to find the house cell phone.

I reached up and pulled a few squares of toilet paper. The fall hadn't felt that serious, but what did I know? I felt around for the gash with the toilet paper. I imagined squiggly gray brain matter oozing from my skull. I took a deep breath before looking at the wadded tissue. Blood definitely, but not copious amounts. No signs of brain.

David came back in with the phone, and I said, "Try to call your dad."

No parent wants a phone call from their adult child in the middle of the night, but Dr. Dave handled it like a champ, thanks to decades of on-call nights as a family physician.

Still on the floor with my head bent between my knees, I flipped through the house manual that David had brought with him from the other room. All restaurant and beach suggestions—nothing helpful. I kept my mouth shut.

Such an idiot, I berated myself. *How can you be so clumsy? And not knowing a number to call in an emergency is unforgivable! Poor David.*

Above my head, Dr. Dave assured David that I was likely okay, that a concussion was not likely in that part of the skull, and I didn't need stitches because the bleeding stopped when he applied pressure.

We made our way back to the bedroom and lay quietly together. The room and the sounds were the same as before I fell: the gentle sound of the waves crashing, the breeze blowing into our room.

But *we* were suddenly very different.

❧

I swam one more time, after all.

We drove down to the southern tip of the island where the cruise ship terminal (complete with Margaritaville Grand Turk) had claimed the best beach as its own. The massive ship in port blocked the view of the Caribbean but also the choppiness of the waves. David, worried that I would go under again, held me in his arms most of the time. We blended in quite nicely, our bodies entwined. Although, I was quite sure we were the most miserable couple on the beach.

For the rest of the week, we chose remote beaches. We sat side-by-side on the sand for hours and watched the relentless change of the ocean. When my yearning to swim in the impossibly blue water welled up so viciously that I wiped away a tear, David wrapped his arm around my shoulders. He reminded me that it was thirty degrees at home in Maryland.

I laughed and leaned into him a little harder.

Staring out into the water, I imagined the life and death struggles taking place—right now—under the surface. Struggles no one would witness except the predator and the prey, so they meant nothing and everything all at once to the evolution of life. My mind flicked back to the conundrum about cremation. *It's the same. If I am cremated and scattered, there will be nothing left of me.* But the prey that is eaten nourishes the predator. When the predator dies, its flesh and bones nourish someone else—a larger predator, a scavenger, plankton.

Life is so temporary.

But it always continues.

If my ashes were scattered here, in the Caribbean, I would go on to nourish other life. Maybe a speck of me would become a shark. A speck of me would become a shell. Or a fish. *Think of all the adventures I would have!*

I laughed out loud. Decision made.

⥥

Aside from sitting on the beach, we spent most of the week hanging out on the porch of the little rental house, facing the water, reading. From the bookshelf, David picked up a dog-eared copy of *The Kite Runner*, which he'd never read but was one of my all-time favorite books. I asked him hourly for an update of what was going on with Amir, Hassan, and Baba.

I rotated between *Wild* by Cheryl Strayed and Dr. Brené Brown's *The Gifts of Imperfection*, depending on my mood.

I turned to *The Gifts of Imperfection*. I suppressed an eye roll at the title. *If Dr. Brown only knew how "imperfect" a life could turn in a matter of months*, I thought. Perhaps: *The Other Shoe Has Officially Dropped* would be a better title. But the "gifts" of imperfection? Oh, come on.

And of course, in the way that only Dr. Brown can do, she encouraged me to reframe the narrative I'd been telling myself. Learning to embrace the journey our lives—in all of its imperfection—*is* the gift. When we become that brave, it doesn't matter how many shoes drop (or get thrown at us).

I swallowed hard. She was talking about Acceptance. I would try to own my story—and love myself through it. And, I guess, that meant I would be brave, too. I was willing to try.

CHAPTER 16

THE BRIGHT LINE
OF COMMUNITY

January 2015

My triathlon finish convinced a couple of my friends to sign up for their own races. Carissa: her first half marathon. Molly: her first IRONMAN.

Jon Blais had inspired me, then I did something—initially to inspire myself—that ended up inspiring others. I loved that. I felt a bright line of inspiration stretching between Jon's legacy and myself, and now to my friends.

I so clearly remembered my first half marathon, marathon, and half-distance triathlon before I was diagnosed. And then, of course, the most extraordinary experience of the post-diagnosis Ramblin' Rose triathlon.

Everyone should have that feeling of invincibility at least once in their lives, I thought.

What if I challenged more people to do a race of their own? And what if this challenge also raised money for ALS research? I remember how my heart soared with every donation—it wasn't just the money; it was the feeling of my friends and family supporting me.

The race distance didn't matter—only that it represented a personal challenge to the individual. Then, maybe for the first time ever, they would experience that glorious finish line feeling!

I had no clue how many people would take on a challenge like this. But even twenty people each raising $250 would result in $5,000 raised for the Blazeman Foundation.

I grew more excited about the possibilities and promptly got to work convincing others to accept the Team Drea Challenge. I posted:

> There is no feeling in the world like the moment you cross the finish line of a race you've worked so hard for and weren't at all sure you could finish. But the best part is looking back and realizing it was really the daily grind of training, staying committed, overcoming setbacks, prioritizing your health, breathing hard, pushing through, sweating and just being alive—the journey itself—that was actually the reward all along. That post-race high can be just enough to crack open your accepted image of yourself (with all your self-imposed limitations) to see your life and its possibilities differently.

Within a month, forty people signed up.

I was stunned. Another spark ignited—no, *forty* more sparks!

While I assumed that people would sign up for all sorts of race events, my community surprised me with their creativity and ambition. Carrie committed to a 5K ninja obstacle race as her first race ever. Ashley and Doug planned to run one event per month *and* push their children in a double stroller. My friend Lauran in Scotland mapped out fifteen different races—the total distances adding up to 179 miles.

We aimed to raise $10,000 for ALS research, which was incredible.

More incredible was the potential impact. Because my friends all had friends, we could reach more people. That bright line stretching from Jon Blais to me could now extend even farther, reaching out in countless directions like rays of sunshine. Our goal to help find a cure for ALS would also change as many lives as we could in the process.

If we could accomplish these things?

Then my ALS would result in something positive in the world.

August 2015

Funny how things happen. The Team Drea Challenge I created to inspire others ended up inspiring *me*.

Even a year after my ALS diagnosis, my body hadn't failed—which felt like reason enough to celebrate—and to keep triking.

One hot, late summer afternoon, I had the entire trail to myself. Well, almost. My mood took a dive the moment I spotted *her*.

For the most part, I could now see a runner and not burst into tears (that had taken some work). But I still ached with a wound that would never quite heal. The wound of ALS. The wound of never being able to run again.

Watching her calf and thigh muscles tensing, arms pumping, and her ponytail swinging triggered the ache. She wore an orange tank top and fitted black shorts showing off a cute figure. I wore a shapeless T-shirt and mesh shorts.

Envy churned inside my head. *That should be ME.*

I followed her, even though I knew I was just torturing myself, and for no good reason.

But I couldn't help it. I followed her on my trike and stared.

Her foot pushed off the ground. For a split second, she was airborne as her hip, knee, and ankle drove forward, carrying the other foot effortlessly through stride. Her heel hit the asphalt at the exact, precise angle, then rolled through her stride. *Push, drive, carry, land, push, drive, carry, land.* A glorious, well-programmed machine in motion. And she wasn't thinking about any of it. She was listening to her headphones.

Running was automatic. Her motor neurons fired on their own. Her muscle fibers strained and relaxed normally. She swung her perfect ponytail, listened to music as her perfect neurological glue held her together. *That should be ME!*

Knowing full well I was driving myself into a wild rage, I hunted her down with uneven pedal strokes as my legs shook uncontrollably. My little green trike bounced over tree roots in the trail that jiggled my body mercilessly.

She turned down an unpaved path I could not follow.

I clenched my brakes, slowed to a stop, and watched her disappear down the trail. A small whimper escaped with my exhale. *That should be me.*

I closed my eyes to keep the tears from coming. When I opened them, I realized the light on the trail had changed. The shadows had taken over. A darkness hung in the air. I sighed and began pedaling again.

The ability to be using your muscles in any form is a gift. If you had a fast-progressing form of ALS, you would be dead by now. My inner-dialogue pep talk was speaking facts.

But I couldn't help feeling crushed. My entire life had changed in a year—literally everything. *Also facts.*

In March, I'd finally stopped working. I traded my hard-won career for disability benefits. I no longer required a career anyway because my *new* job was learning how to die.

But even that was winding down: I finished my will, indexed all the photos, recorded a video for my funeral, and now waited for my body to fail me. And yet, it hadn't. My body was still responding to my brain—slowly.

Before ALS, I tried to keep up with faster runners or pass the slower ones. I had been competitive, and chasing Orange Tank Top made me realize that I was still competitive. Maybe I needed competition—even if the competition was with myself. To see what I could do.

To my left was a wide street with a long incline. The hill looked quite steep—but also doable. *Well, that hill looks like a competition.*

Changing gears, I dialed in my focus. I cranked up the hill, using the entire pedal stroke to press through my quads and pull up with my feet. My pace was slow—anyone out for a casual walk would have passed me. But I was working hard. It felt good. *This does not feel like dying.*

Pedal by pedal, I made it up the hill. Sweating, breathing hard, and happy.

In creating the Team Drea Challenge for others, I assumed my racing days were behind me. I wanted others to pick a big goal. To do something so big that it scared them. That was the point: stretch, reach, be brave.

But after climbing that hill, I thought, *What if there are more races ahead—for me?*

On the way back down the hill, I let myself fly. As the trike picked up speed, I smiled and leaned into the wind. Faster and faster until the houses streaking by became a blur. *Why have I never done this before?*

By the time I reached the bottom of the hill, I made a promise to myself. I decided to live bravely—not to just ask others to do it.

I would sign up for a full marathon on my trike.

What's the worst that can happen? I thought. *I crash and die? Big deal. That is going to happen anyway.*

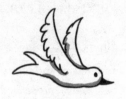

CHAPTER 17

A FIRST MARATHON

North Carolina: Marathon #1

True to my word, I signed up for the City of Oaks Marathon in my hometown of Raleigh, North Carolina. Two years earlier, that relay convinced me to see a PT about my tight hamstrings and balance problems.

Training for a marathon was one thing. But sixty friends, spouses, and children were coming for the Team Drea Halloween weekend costume party *and* to race. That was quite another thing entirely (ahem, let's remember my wedding).

The party was a thank-you for not only the fundraising and generosity of Team Drea, but also the gifts of purpose and community my friends had given me. Team Drea tethered me to *life*—where people had goals and were *living*, rather than merely staving off death.

The year before had been filled with uncertainty and dread. This year had been life-affirming. Coming from a dying woman, that's saying something. *How do I adequately thank my friends for giving me purpose, community, and life?* The pressure felt enormous.

So I did what I usually did under pressure. I freaked out.

The catering, the venue, the party favors, the never-ending list of details. Just like a wedding, only I could no longer move as fast or speak with enough clarity to delegate. I couldn't stop the tentacles of anxiety from rising—threatening to choke me.

Consistent positivity in the face of death is not for the faint of heart.

The words I spoke constantly: *our precious time is short; how lucky we are to be able to come together; how lucky I am to still be alive; blah blah blah blah* . . . I believed them, but they weren't enough to negate my frustrating reality: I couldn't do anything fast enough.

By the time David and I left at 4 A.M. to make the drive from Maryland to North Carolina, I was exhausted. Ready to snap. As we pulled into the venue—a public park—the lot was already full.

"Where are people going to *park*?" I wailed as David circled.

David, who had been living with my freak-outs for a week now (*years*, if we're honest), shot me a look.

"People will figure it out," he said.

The venue was perfect: a patio overlooking the lake, reflecting the autumn beauty of the turning leaves. A cozy room for lunch. Charming rocking chairs.

But the anxiety tentacles tightened their grip as David and my parents unloaded party supplies. I could do nothing but sit, kneading my hands, stressed out by all the things I couldn't do.

Once inside, everyone started firing questions at me about favors and tables and seating. I froze.

David took one look at my face and took charge. Orders issued, he motioned me outside.

"Are you okay?" he asked.

He wasn't really asking. His tone had a warning in it.

I closed my eyes, frustrated, my face scrunching. *I should be happy. I should be grateful. But I am just so pissed. I can't talk fast enough or loud enough to be useful. I can't do anything.*

David's expression didn't soften, even when I crumpled.

"You need to pull it together, babe. You are stronger than this."

I looked up at him and straightened my weary spine. He was my person. He knew exactly what to say to me. I wanted to believe him, even if I wasn't sure I did. But I knew I wouldn't let him down.

"Okay." I exhaled deeply.

The party was on—full of friends wearing costumes ranging from banana bread* (that would be David) to bumblebee. By the time the icebreaker game—Team Drea Bingo—was in full swing, I had regained perspective. Looking around the party, I allowed myself to be proud.

My original thought was that we would raise $5,000 for research. Then $10,000. But our fifty members had raised over $80,000 for ALS research through the Blazeman Foundation.

At the end of the party, we all gathered by the railing overlooking the lake. I pulled out a small Ziploc bag Jon's parents had sent me.

Jon Blais's final wish was to be taken to beautiful places he would never see because of the time—and life—ALS took from him.

I had spread some of his ashes once before.

Six months earlier, David and I had participated in the Blazeman 5K in Jon's home state of Rhode Island, where I met his parents, Bob and Mary Ann, for the first time.

Mary Ann Blais greeted us with a big smile and hug, but her eyes seemed to hold a permanent sadness. We had become close over emails and phone calls in the previous few months. I could tell that seeing a future ALS victim standing in front of her was a tough reminder for her.

Bob Blais, however, was a force of joy. His white mustache danced as he introduced me to everyone he could find. He was surrounded by people who loved Jon and his mission. And that brought him happiness.

"Before we start the race," Bob said to me, "will you do the honors of spreading Jon's ashes at the start line?"

"Of course." *What else could I say?* Like his parents, I would have done anything for Jon—the person who had inspired me to get the trike for one last race.

But holding mixed-and-matched bits of his cremated body? It struck me as too much like a front row seat to my own future. *Maybe I just won't look . . .*

Bob gathered the crowd at the start line. He spoke about Jon, his legacy, the war on ALS, and the power of community. Then it was time for the ceremony.

---

* An homage to Ashley, who had baked fifty loaves of banana bread that I mailed out in care packages before everyone's races.

Seated in my trike under a magnificent old oak tree, with David's hand on my shoulder, I remembered the peace I felt on the beach in Turks and Caicos. About my own future. About how a speck of me would become a shark or a shell. I pictured the new adventures Jon would go on by the spreading of his ashes.

I leaned over the side of the trike and opened the plastic bag.

As I scattered Jon beneath the tree, an honest, pure curiosity took over. I didn't close my eyes. I saw the bits of bone mixed within a grayish white powder. That was all. Ashes to ashes.

My anxiety gave way to a deep understanding and *knowing*.

We as a crowd, collectively, breathed *in* oxygen under that tree. We, collectively, breathed *out* carbon dioxide. Jon's ashes would mix into the soil and nourish the ground, the oak tree. The oak tree would give off oxygen, grow leaves, lose leaves, and . . . on and on. The air, the tree, the bits of bone, every one of us in the crowd: it was all just *life*. Life begets life.

At the Team Drea party, I carefully sprinkled more of Jon into the water. *Time for a new adventure, Jon. Thank you for inspiring us.*

Jon's inspiration lives on through everyone who has heard his story, who has done a Blazeman Roll. He inspired me, I inspired Team Drea, and on and on. Inspiration begets inspiration.

❦

Twenty-two Team Drea runners scattered throughout the course for the marathon relay to run alongside me at various points. Or they were at the start line for their own half marathons. I was the only one racing for Team Drea who had signed up for the full marathon.

My second marathon ever.

The first in my trike.

Honestly, compared to party planning, pedaling for several hours in a straight line seemed downright easy. No organizing, no coordinating, no questions, very little talking. Just pedaling and hanging out with the friends I loved so much. Maybe that's why I forgot to feel nervous that I was doing a *marathon*.

Amy and Jodi ran the first leg with me. They had come into my life thanks to that last triathlon. Amy was the race director for Ramblin' Rose, and Jodi had read the article that appeared in *Endurance* magazine about the race.

Above my helmeted head, they bonded over that story and the other things they discovered they had in common: raising three kids, running the Chicago Marathon, and how they still missed the mothers they'd lost—one to cancer, one to ALS. Running helped them process, grieve, and keep on living.

On the second leg, I triked beside Jodi's sister, Jillaine. Two years (and a lifetime) ago, I had run part of this race as a relay—on my own two feet. I had walked all the downhills because I was tripping over my toes. *My last run ever.*

On the third leg, I picked up my friend Carrie. Her Team Drea race, a ninja 5K obstacle course, had been more ambitious than she'd realized. She took her challenge seriously, though, and hired a personal trainer and a nutritionist. The nutritionist discovered that Carrie had a gluten intolerance. After some dietary modifications, Carrie began to feel better than she had in decades.

The fourth and final leg was with David and Julie. Just like at Ramblin' Rose, we three would cross the finish line together.

For the first time all day, I struggled.

The fourth leg of the race was all up, up, up. I huffed and puffed, grinding up the hills. But slowly, the trike came to a stop. I just didn't have the strength or momentum to push one foot over the other. I clamped on the brakes so I didn't roll backward. I tried to catch my breath.

"Do you want a push?" David asked. I gulped air and considered. *It's not like I have a choice here.* I couldn't do it on my own, as much as I wanted to. *Accept help, Andrea.*

Seconds later, David was the one huffing and puffing. I churned my legs to help. Julie walked beside us.

About a hundred yards from the finish line, I saw Team Drea clustered on the sidewalk, waiting and cheering. They spilled out into the street, from all corners of my life.

We crossed the finish line together—a beautiful foreshadowing of something I hadn't even dreamed about yet.

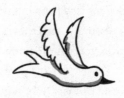

CHAPTER 18

HOPE GETS SCRAPPY

January 2016

Although I remained careful to skip over emotionally charged posts, the online ALS community provided a wealth of information. From health to relationships to end of life, no question is off-limits for discussion in an online ALS forum.

But the most popular subject, by far, is *poop*.

Questions about the feeding tube and its required liquid diet causing poop issues. The side effects of medications that cause problems with poop. Caregivers ask which adult diapers are best for their bedridden loved ones, which bidet to buy, and the best technique for helping someone use the bathroom from a Hoyer lift (basically, a human sling) suspended over the toilet. More questions about urgency, travel, and stool softeners.

I had poop questions, too—mostly fears. How could I endure such a mortifying loss of independence? Needing to use the bathroom—each time—with assistance? Since my diagnosis, I had been borderline panicking about the topic of poop.

Constipated was a great word for this time in my life, actually.

As my muscles became increasingly stiff, they also weakened. As a result, I spent more time in the bathroom, trying to poop with my increasingly stiff, increasingly weak muscles.

Since my diagnosis, I had been carrying around another type of impaction, if you will: the idea of my entire life, completely derailed. My future reeked of medical appointments, clinical trials, and wheelchairs, packed in by assisted bathroom trips and the general dirty work of dying. No wonder I felt bloated and irritable.

The marathon, well, flushed me out in ways I hadn't expected.

In the weeks following the race, I felt lighter, healthier, and more like myself than I had in a long time. This afterglow felt different from the triathlon I'd finished with Julie and David by my side. I had been riding with friends and training for almost a year leading up to the marathon. I felt muscles in my legs that weren't there before.

Hadn't been there, in fact, since the neurologists advised me *not* to exercise while they figured out what was wrong with me. I listened to their advice and stopped moving, waiting for a diagnosis. I dared not move, for fear of what movement might do to me.

And for what? In that short period of time—from the first neurologist to a probable ALS diagnosis—I had declined from the strongest I'd ever been to walking with a cane. Four months. What a waste. *Never again,* I thought.

Over and over, I repeated those words: *never again.*

Whatever the (conflicting) medical literature said about exercise and ALS, whatever the doctors told me, whatever cautionary tales I read online—I needed to let it all wash over me like impenetrable waves. *Never again.* In the sea of ALS uncertainty, I began to trust my inner knowing: I could navigate better with movement. I knew something different because I had experienced something different.

The "brand" of ALS in my body responded to slow, focused, muscle-building exercises. I added in extra sleep and lowered my day-to-day stress.

Riding my trike became the perfect addition to my healthy plan. Not only did I love my little green trike—I *needed* it. My body needed the exercise, the goals, and that glorious feeling of freedom.

My inner knowing spoke up clearly: *I am tired of waiting around for this disease to kill me. I'm just going to do whatever I want, until I can't do it anymore.*

(Not) surprisingly, what I wanted? More marathons.

But as I searched for more marathons, I learned something new. No marathons had a category for recumbent trikes.

All marathons allowed push-rim wheelchairs. Some allowed handcycles. I had tried the handcycle, but my upper body was too weak for long distances. I could barely make it two miles on flat ground—if a hill was involved, forget it. Maybe I could get strong enough to use one, but that would take years, and hell, I'd probably be dead by then.

My power was my legs. That's how *my* ALS worked.

I fired off emails to race directors, explaining my situation and requesting permission to participate on my trike.

> *I have ALS (Lou Gehrig's disease) and can no longer run, but I finished a marathon in Raleigh last November with a time of 4:53 on a recumbent trike. I need no special assistance on race courses, and I will have friends running with me or nearby just in case. I would love to participate in your race. Please let me know if this would be allowed.*

A few race directors wrote back: "Yes! We would be honored to have you." But most said no.

Some had good reasons: the race took place on a narrow trail with traffic in two directions, or parts of the race were off-road—those reasons made perfect sense to me. I couldn't handle the trike on those courses anyway.

However, others seemed flippant:

"We only allow racing wheelchairs, no handcycles." *A trike isn't a handcycle.*

"Our insurance won't allow it." *Did you check? I emailed you only ten minutes ago.*

One race required permission from USA Track & Field (USATF), the review of which was delayed by the Olympic trials. *Hold up, the same committee that makes decisions for the Olympics needed to review my request for a tiny race in New York?*

The denials not based on legitimate safety concerns smacked of discrimination. The Americans with Disabilities Act (ADA) ensures "reasonable accommodations" for people with disabilities. I just wanted to participate in road races in the only way I was able, given my disabilities—on my trike.

I came to learn why race directors balked at introducing an unfamiliar adaptive vehicle like my trike into their events. And it had nothing to do with me.

As with most instances of systemic inequality, history tells the true story.

The push-rim wheelchair was the first adaptive vehicle used in an official event, in the 1964 Tokyo Paralympics.[1] Athletes who couldn't run due to spinal cord injuries or amputations used their hands to grab wheel rims and propel themselves forward: no gears, just tremendous upper body strength. Over time, racing wheelchairs evolved to include a third wheel in front, increasing stability and aerodynamics.

Next, the handcycle emerged with a wave of controversy. Unlike a racing wheelchair, a handcycle has gears to make hill climbing easier. The handcycle helped athletes with less upper body strength or who couldn't handle a push-rim wheelchair.

A handcyclist with no upper body limitations, however, can go *very* fast.

Some handcyclists were so fast, they'd get out in front of the lead pace car, police, and road closures, essentially riding in open traffic—a race director's nightmare.

The push-rim wheelchair versus handcycle debate made it to the media and the courtroom. Push-rim proponents argued that the handcycle was unsafe and unfair with its gears. Handcycle proponents countered that the wheelchair riders were just tired of getting beat. There was definite gray area. Wheelchair racers and handcyclists took digs at each other in news articles.[2] Lawsuits were filed and settled.[3]

I wasn't on either side of this debate. I had a different set of physical issues and a different adaptation. I was hardly in danger of getting ahead of *any* race and causing safety issues. My marathon pace, at this time, was around an eleven-minute mile—which is basically a jog for a marathoner on foot.

I didn't have time—literally or figuratively—for debates and lawsuits.

I just wanted to do more marathons, in the only way I could—on my trike.

Racing was only part of the goal, anyway. I also wanted to write. I wanted to dedicate each race to someone *living* with ALS and write about it for social media. Maybe I could weave the stories into a book one day. The ALS memoir *I* wanted to read.

Typical ALS memoirs are brutal, no matter how beautifully they are written. The plot is always the same: the person with ALS comes to terms with their death, finds happiness anyway—or at least peace—even though all hope is lost.

The horrific nature of ALS is important for people outside of the disease to understand. And certainly therapeutic for the writer. But if you are already living through the nightmare of ALS, reading about it is doubly rough.

Take, for example, Jenifer Estess's 2004 memoir, *Tales from the Bed*. She was diagnosed at age thirty-five, close to my age. She and I had similar winding paths toward diagnosis. Reading about her commitment to raising money for research through Project ALS, I bonded with her through her powerful words on the page.

But I got too close.

I already knew the inevitable and tragic end to Jenifer's story. Like a friend, I loved her too much to want to let her go. I read slower as the disease took control of her body, dreading what was coming in the remaining pages. I had finally found someone who understood me, and I was losing her.

Just like Darcy Wakefield in *I Remember Running*, a book I forced myself to finish months ago. Tales of strong women, focused on fulfilling their life's purpose, and just when things were starting to get good—*BAM!* They died. Even the writing fell off in later chapters as the disease took over.

I needed some friends with ALS who weren't dead writers. Friends my own age, fighting the same fight. Friends I didn't have to say goodbye to when they died at the end of the book.

I *had* started meeting people with ALS doing all sorts of cool stuff with their remaining days. In fact, dying pushed them to pursue more interesting and meaningful lives. I wanted to learn from them.

So that became my plan: race in honor of people living with ALS and then write about them—and, perhaps, how they found their own versions of Hope.

Naturally, I started with the guy who stole the doughnut truck.

Chris Rosati was diagnosed with ALS at thirty-nine. His wife was five months pregnant with their second child. He experienced his first muscle twitches when training for a triathlon and started his own medical mystery tour when he could no longer open a jar.

Chris was a vice president of marketing for a healthcare company. He continued in his job for another two years but became increasingly restless. Colleagues raised their eyebrows and exchanged looks whenever Chris walked out of a meeting he deemed a waste of time.

One day, he simply quit.

When his high school alma mater invited him to give a talk, Chris spoke sincerely from the heart about his greatest regret: worrying too much. And then he told the students a recurring dream—to steal a Krispy Kreme doughnut truck and take it on a joyride, giving away doughnuts like Robin Hood.

Apparently, "You can't tell four hundred high school kids that you're really happy you tried in your life, and then tell them about the Krispy Kreme thing and then not try to do it," he later told the local paper.[4]

When he posted his idea on social media, Krispy Kreme offered up a bus stocked with doughnuts. Chris, his family, and friends drove around all day, handing out doughnuts at city parks, cancer wards, the children's hospital, even at his old high school.

"Chris says if dying has taught him anything, it's about how to live. He says you have to do what you can to make people smile while you still have the chance," CBS News reported.[5]

Capitalizing on the media attention, Chris created a nonprofit organization, Inspire MEdia, with Krispy Kreme as a key donor. He launched the BIGG (Big Idea for the Greater Good) initiative to encourage young people to submit their "most creative, bold and uncommon ways to enrich the lives of others." Inspire MEdia picked the winners, the students filmed themselves carrying out their ideas, and held a red-carpet event to show the results. Winning ideas included setting up a booth for adults to color like kids and inviting homeless strangers to a fancy dinner. Chris planned to package the content and sell it to media outlets.

Chris certainly inspired *me*. His accomplishments weren't in spite of his disease, but rather, ALS was the backdrop for his story. ALS set the stage, and Chris poured in his creative vision and marketing genius. The Krispy Kreme heist wasn't a publicity stunt designed to get attention for a product, a company, or even Chris himself. The goal was to spread kindness. And the realization that a dying man was behind the stunt sent the story viral and touched people deeply.

"If I can't impact people, this whole [ALS] thing is a waste," Chris told CBS.

⌘

Initially, I had wanted to do twelve marathons in twelve months, but I couldn't find enough marathons that would let me in. So instead, I completed a mix of twelve races in 2016: three marathons, eight half marathons, and one triathlon. I loved racing, of course, but honestly, was more thrilled to meet and write about so many interesting people with ALS and their own unique versions of Hope:

- Beth Hebron posed as the "Styled Mannequin" in artsy, elaborate social media shoots. This was quite a feat, considering she was almost paralyzed.
- Mickey Johnston, a.k.a. "Shy Tuna," mailed out 450 tie-dyed shirts to people with ALS to make them smile.
- Steve Dezember created gorgeous works of art by driving his power wheelchair into paint—and then over a canvas.
- Matt Bellina, a former Air Force pilot, led the Right to Try legislative movement to encourage pharmaceutical companies to grant early access to clinical trial drugs.
- Arthur Cohen became the chief pickle officer of the nonprofit pickle-making company PickALS, based on the recipe his friends and family loved.
- Amanda Bernier, a thirty-year-old firefighter with familial ALS, was diagnosed two weeks after finding out she was pregnant. She was paralyzed by the time her baby was born, yet she insisted on breastfeeding—and created scrapbooks, journals, cards, and Christmas gifts for her daughter to open over the next twenty-one years.

- Sarah Coglianese wrote stunningly real and raw blog posts—which had me alternatively laughing and crying.
- Augie Nieto, the founder of LifeFitness workout equipment and Augie's Quest, which has raised $88 million for ALS research, lived for eighteen years with the disease.
- And Mayuri Saxena . . . her story comes later.

With each race I finished and each story I wrote, I learned more about Hope. I learned how to create a life of purpose and meaning, even in the face of death. All these people had found Hope in their own way. They knew they didn't have long to make a difference, to make art, or to impact their communities. But they went for it anyway.

It felt . . . *scrappy*.

I wanted to be all about the same scrappy Hope and to offer inspiration to others. By the end of 2016, I definitely felt I was on my way. I had finished marathons and triathlons with ALS, created the new Team Drea Foundation (an official nonprofit), and had raised $200,000 for ALS research.

Like the sun breaking through the clouds after a storm, the Hope inside of me wanted to shine. Hope became the voice of the strong woman within, pushing me to see what else I could do.

CHAPTER 19

THE EVER-FUCKING-PRACTICAL LISA

Virginia: Marathon #2

In March 2016, I took on the Yuengling Shamrock Marathon in Virginia Beach on my trike in memory of my first "in real life" ALS friend, Lisa.

I ran that same race as my first marathon back in 2012. The only full marathon I had—or would ever—run on my own two feet.

When I created the Team Drea Challenge, the 2012 Shamrock Marathon was the finish line I pictured. It cracked open my self-imposed limitations of what I could accomplish. The finish line photo captured me fist-pumping the air, tears of joy hidden behind my sunglasses. The feeling was so transformational and addictive that I wanted to keep racing forever.

Returning on my trike in 2016, I carried no illusions about the inevitability of future races—nor my own invincibility. I would celebrate each finish line as its own accomplishment.

But so much for my plan to write about people *living* with ALS—the disease is so fucking relentless that it stole Lisa away just as our friendship was getting good.

I didn't know what else to do with my grief and survivor's guilt—except a marathon for Lisa.

February 2015

Lisa McMillen was diagnosed just before her thirty-first birthday in April 2014, only a month before I learned of my probable ALS. A social worker at the ALS Clinic connected us. We lived close to each other, so David and I planned an adult playdate to meet Lisa and her husband, Sean.

Considering Lisa and I had basically the same ALS "starting line," I assumed we'd be at the same stage of ALS.

I was wrong. And in disbelief when the door opened.

Lisa was beautiful and exquisitely dressed. She had curly, dark hair falling around her shoulders. But my eyes locked onto her wheelchair, and on the one shaky finger she stretched out to touch my hand in greeting.

I swallowed hard and smiled. Then I awkwardly hugged the back of her enormous wheelchair, not sure how to execute a proper hug under these circumstances.

I could not understand her words. Thankfully, Sean translated Lisa's speech for us. I *hated* that I couldn't understand her because I *hated* when people couldn't understand me.

Lisa, through Sean, said that my diagnosis story was awful—way worse than hers. I argued that she had the worst story. This is the odd ALS-type banter you get into when you're in the shitty ALS club.

Lisa had a stroke as a teenager, so when a second incident occurred when Lisa and Sean were newlyweds, the doctors assumed a second stroke. She spent a long time in the hospital. Her twin sister Kat, a neurological PT at the same hospital, and their mom, Angela, had Lisa's bathroom remodeled with a roll-in shower. With Sean, they prepared for a long rehabilitation.

But her symptoms kept getting worse. Months of collective medical head scratching went on: the same tests with needles and electrodes, referrals to new doctors, and the same frustration David and I experienced.

Lisa finally received the dreaded diagnosis of ALS that Kat had suspected for months.

We laughed about the similarities in our husbands. Both attorneys, both grew up outside Philly, both rowed in college. Sean also looked at Lisa the same way that David looked at me. Sean would do anything for Lisa . . . and basically *was* doing everything for her.

He spoon-fed each bite of her soup. (She couldn't lift her arms.) He instinctively kept an eye on the straw in her glass of wine and seamlessly moved it closer if she had trouble reaching it with her mouth. (She couldn't lean too far forward.) He wiped her mouth every few minutes. (She would occasionally drool.)

I watched Sean and Lisa carefully. I felt the love between them. But I also felt a dark foreboding rolling in. In a few years (months?), that would be David and me.

Outwardly, we maintained a spirited conversation with our new friends. But I could barely eat. My insides were crawling, screaming and revolting in abject fear. The ALS elephant in the room was big and loud and scary.

Through Sean, Lisa told us that even though she could still eat, she opted to have a feeding tube put in early, when her body was at its strongest. She was so matter-of-fact and practical about everything. She wasn't depressed or wallowing in self-pity about what she couldn't do, which was a lot less than I still could.

"You just have to stay ahead of this disease," she said. The repeated line from the ALS Clinic meant more coming from Lisa.

Lisa and Sean lived in a daylight basement condo, which had four steps up to ground level. Lisa pushed a button on the remote control sitting on her lap and the front door swung open. She navigated her power chair onto a giant beige box of a platform lift that she could operate from a close-to-her-hand switch on a wall inside the lift.

I pictured our house—the one we'd just bought nine months ago.

We had about the same number of steps, but our house was at grade. Which means that if I needed a lift, we'd have to install the large bland beige box outside our front door. No way to hide it. *Ugh.* I hated the idea of announcing to each passerby exactly what I could no longer do.

Sean and Lisa's accessible minivan was also a bland beige box.

"It's nothing to look at, but it does the job," Sean said, pushing the button to unfold the automatic ramp.

At this point, Lisa insisted I drive her power wheelchair.

Despite the cold weather, my skin broke out in a mild sweat. *No. No. No.* I protested, lightly, then more firmly. I really, really wasn't ready for the power chair. I wasn't ready to imagine my future, let alone sit in it. *No. No. No.*

"No, really, I'd rather not," I said.

"It's okay," Lisa said, catching my expression. "I said no to it for a long time."

"But it was so much better after you started using it, right, babe?" Sean chimed in. Lisa nodded. I couldn't look at David.

I didn't want to be rude to our hosts, or make Lisa think there was something wrong with using a wheelchair. *No. No. No.* So I reluctantly agreed.

Sean pulled a folding wheelchair out of the back of the minivan. David and I silently watched Sean scoop Lisa out of her power chair and place her gently into the other wheelchair. She couldn't have weighed more than ninety pounds.

David helped me climb into the black leather chair. I put my hand down in the center of the seat to find some leverage to adjust myself. The cushion wheezed like an air mattress deflating. I pulled my hand away, alarmed.

"Oh, don't worry about that," Sean said. "It's filled with air so you don't get pressure sores from sitting all day, every day." *No. No. No.*

"Okay," I said, shooting a look at David that I hoped Sean and Lisa couldn't see.

Sean taught me how to drive. A little joystick at the end of the right armrest controlled the steering. A screen at the end of the left armrest controlled the speed, adjusted the backrest, and raised the footrests. The chair even had an elevator-type feature—to raise its rider to talk to someone at eye level or reach a plate or glass in a cabinet. Well, assuming the rider could still raise their arms and had fingers that could grasp dishes.

Had I not been so horrified by the glimpse into my future, I would have been impressed by the chair.

I did a few loops in the parking lot. But this chair was nothing like driving my adorable green trike for the first time. I tried to smile as I drove toward the others, but when I navigated in the other direction, I struggled mightily to hold back the tears. *This cannot be my future.*

"It's really cool," I said when I finished my test drive.

"It just allows you so much freedom," Lisa said (through Sean).

Freedom. Not the word I would have chosen.

Even though the first visit was tough, Lisa and I became tight. We texted regularly—we would have been friends even without ALS. She was funny and sweet, and used as many emojis as I did. I was no longer freaked about her ALS devices and the progression of her illness. And since I had awkwardly test-driven her wheelchair on our first visit, that was now out of the way and we could get on with our friendship.

Naturally, most of our texted conversations revolved around ALS. I could complain to her about how depressing ALS Clinic was. She understood because she endured it too.

"They keep talking about things I don't need yet," I said.

"Like what?" she asked. "I realllllly resisted the wheelchair talk."

"Wheelchair, even though I walk okay with a walker. Not driving, even though I drive fine. Feeding tube, even though I'm only having trouble with water."

"Did they send you to NRH for a driving evaluation?" she asked, referring to the National Rehabilitation Hospital in DC, where I was still going for physical therapy twice a week.

"No."

"That was why I had to stop driving . . . my hand and foot were bad."

"David was actually the one who brought it up. I was so mad at him. I was like, what do I have to do to prove it to you? You drive with me ALL the time. But he was just worrying about being the one who would have to take the keys away from me."

"Would the evaluation help him leave you alone? I'll give you the info!"

Lisa was just so damn practical.

One day at lunch with Lisa and her mom, Angela, I learned exactly why Lisa had stopped going into the office for work. In the bathroom, she had fallen *inside* the locked stall. She was wearing a dress but her underwear was down. One of her colleagues crawled under the stall door to unlock it.

I was appropriately sympathetic without saying "how mortifying!" which was really what I was thinking. The underwear down plus pickup by a work colleague was way worse than falling in the lobby of my new office building.

That was the thing about ALS: it was always—and only—going to get worse.

And that was the last time I saw Lisa.

Lisa died on May 15, 2015, two days after her (and Kat's) thirty-second birthday. I had sent her a birthday text but received no response. I knew she wasn't doing well. A week before she died, a mutual friend confided that her breathing was down to 21 percent.

I also knew what happened to people with ALS. They die.

Even knowing that fact, I was shocked by the primal rage that consumed me after she died. I paced around the house with tears streaming down my face, emitting a sound that was closer to a shriek than a wail. *Beautiful, smart, sweet, ever-fucking-practical Lisa!* Trapped inside a failing body with her mind as sharp as ever. Knowing exactly what was happening, and yet being unable to stop it.

I cannot endure that torture. I am not strong enough. I cannot do it. I will just kill myself.

I caught myself instantly. The thought of taking my life shook me harder than Lisa's death. Then I really started to cry. *What is happening to me? Andrea, wake up! No. You don't mean that.*

I didn't mean that. I couldn't do that to David anyway. So instead, I angry-unloaded the dishwasher, slamming the plates and glasses on the counter so hard I thought they would break. *Who cares?* But I realized that sweeping up shards of glass would be difficult for me and might get stuck in little cat paws. *Fucking practical Andrea.*

As pissed off as I was at ALS, I was most mad at myself.

I chose to get close to Lisa, knowing full well that her death was coming. I should have kept my friends limited to dead authors of books. Even worse, though, I was doing the same thing to *my* people all over the world. I was inviting friends to share in my doomed journey via my writing, social media, and Team Drea.

I was forming deep, close friendships and rekindling old ones—and for what? To make it all harder for the people I loved in the end? When I would do the same damn thing that Lisa did? Just up and die!?

Fuck. I stabbed the knives back into their block.

⬥

My cell phone rang a few hours later.

"Hello?"

"Andrea? This is Angela McMillen, Lisa's mom." I froze.

"Hello?" she said.

"I'm-I'm here," I stammered. "Oh . . . I'm so sorry about Lisa's . . . passing." *What an insanely inadequate word.*

"Oh. Thanks," she said, paused, and went on, "Listen, Lisa and I talked about it and we want you to have her van and a bunch of her ALS stuff, okay? We'll set it aside for you."

"Her *van*?" I couldn't believe the generosity. I also couldn't believe I was talking to a mother whose daughter had died fewer than twelve hours prior.

"Yes. The van. Oh, and the automatic door opener. I wish we could get the lift to you. Hmm, actually give me a little time and I'll look into that."

"Oh my goodness. That is so unbelievably gener—"

The quintessential Italian mama, Angela cut me off in such a way that I could picture her flicking her hand. At our last lunch date, Angela had served up steaming bowls of Italian wedding soup and talked almost nonstop. She had an energy and insistence that I knew was very much still on the other end of the phone. I would not protest.

"Lisa made me promise to take care of you, and so that's what I'm going to do. Just let me get some details sorted over the next couple of weeks, and then you and I will go to lunch."

We said goodbye, and I stared at the phone. I smiled my first smile of the day. *Fucking practical Lisa.* Of course she had planned all this.

That night, David came home and wrapped his arms around me. We embraced for a long time. I watched as he pulled down three glasses from the cabinet and filled them with wine. He finished by adding a straw to each, then handed me one for a toast. *Here's to you, Lisa. We poured you one.*

⤚⧓⤙

Now the Shamrock Marathon for Lisa was underway. I smiled for mile after mile, wearing her fleece. Did I feel weird wearing a dead girl's clothes? Strangely, no. Wearing Lisa's clothes covered me in joy, and not just because Lisa had *far* better taste than me. I felt joy bringing her with me during these new adventures.

The weather was yucky: gray sky, forty-four degrees, rain squalls, and gusting wind. *Really, Lisa? You couldn't have dialed up a better forecast for me?*

Nothing with ALS is easy, I could almost hear her say.

Despite the weather, I felt great. Around mile 16, I munched through an entire pack of peanut butter crackers and found myself wondering how I acquired ALS.

Military veterans are twice as likely to be diagnosed with ALS compared to the average population. And then there are the conflicting research studies about exercise. One connecting theory is the greater the stress the human body experiences, the greater susceptibility for ALS.

I knew nothing of nutrition when I ran in the marathon four years earlier. Turns out the average body requires 100–300 calories (ideally, carbohydrates) per hour during a strenuous event. While the exact racing formula varies person to person, suffice it to say I did not come anywhere close to a reasonable, healthy, race-day number of carbohydrates. I had *maybe* consumed 300 calories *total* by hour three. Plus all the months of underfueling during training.

An inadequate nutrition plan likely cannot be blamed for ALS. Long-distance racing with inadequate nutrition likely cannot be blamed for ALS. Military service alone likely cannot be blamed. ALS is more complicated. Even if a physical exertion or nutrition-related link exists, millions of people serve in the military, run marathons, and complete long-distance triathlons without acquiring ALS.

But long-distance racing plus underfueling my training was the only thing I could grasp to blame. Well, I had no one else to blame, right? *Guilty as charged.*

As I pedaled the last miles of the marathon, I turned inward and quietly asked myself forgiveness. *If I brought ALS on myself, I didn't mean to. I didn't know better. I would have never done this intentionally. I just want another chance at life. Please forgive me. Help me forgive myself.*

David met me at mile 23 with pretzels, just as he had in 2012.

I knew he'd be there, but my heart quaked at the sight of him. So much had changed—everything really—except how much I loved David. He was still there, running alongside me all the way to the finish line. Just like Lisa's husband Sean did for her.

2012 Finish Time: 5:15:37
2016 Finish Time: 4:29:18

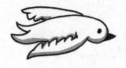

CHAPTER 20

LIAM

August 2015

"Well, it's happened," Lisa had texted me several months before. "Sean finally had to wipe my butt."

The horror I felt reading her words made a decision I'd been deliberating quite easy.

David would eventually wipe my butt, yes. But I could save him from the rest of the "things" in that region. The thought of David removing a bloody tampon and inserting a new one made my skin crawl all the way up to my teeth. *That* issue I could do something about.

I grappled for six months, but finally, on a blistering day in August, I made the decision. I went to my gynecologist for an IUD. The IUD would stop my periods, yes. But it would also stop the possibility of having a baby with David. *That* part cut me to the core.

We hadn't talked about a baby in detail since that first visit to the ALS Clinic, the one where the clinic director stared at me and told me I could be paralyzed by the time I gave birth. Even with that glaring warning, we'd discussed our options on the train ride back to DC.

"I mean, you know my sister would help. She'd love it," David said.

"Yeah, but she was talking about someone *living* with us. She's got her own kids to raise. We can't ask them to do that."

"Yeah," he agreed, his voice trailing off.

"We'd have to move to Philly or Raleigh for our parents to help."

"I can't really see that working out," he said. Neither could I.

After that conversation, we had gone silent on the subject. It had been a year since that visit. In theory, I could have had a baby by now. And I was definitely not paralyzed. *Dammit.*

Driving to the gynecologist's office, I began to have second thoughts about making this decision alone. Not that we had been trying for a baby, but an IUD was taking it a step further. I was closing the door on the possibility. Alone. Talk about guilt.

But if David and I had wanted to figure out how to have a baby, I rationalized to myself, we would have discussed it, right? After all, he knew about the appointment.

All other practical logistics had been covered—in detail. We had discussed the dimensions of renovating the bathroom wide enough for a lift to hoist me in slings onto the toilet. We had discussed end-of-life decisions in completing the will. But for all the hard conversations we had forced ourselves to have, the subject of a baby stayed off-limits. Too painful. The topic hung in the air between us, an unspoken, undiscussed weight on an already heavy marriage. I was making the Acceptance decision for the both of us.

How could I deprive him of such an immeasurable gift, when I had already derailed our life plans so completely? He would be an amazing dad, even if I would probably be dead and gone in one to four years from now, statistically speaking. How selfish was I being?

But seriously, how would having a baby work, Andrea? How could David take care of not one, but two helpless people—the younger of whom would require nighttime feedings and diaper changes, cry relentlessly, and might have health issues of their own, while David held down a full-time demanding job that was solely responsible for our livelihood, did all the shopping, cooking, cleaning, yard work, bill paying, and running of the household entirely on his own?

Not to mention my recurring vision.

In my vision, a cute, chunky-fisted, nursing baby is eating peacefully. David is using this quiet time to grab a shower. I am also somewhat relaxing, the baby against my chest. But then, in a split second, the baby—inadvertently, of course—reaches up and pulls on the breathing apparatus in my nose. Before I know what has happened, the device has come loose. The baby continues to feed, and there I am, unable to lift my arms to reattach my literal lifeline.

That vision made the decision easier for me.

I pulled into the parking deck of the ob-gyn's office. *Still, this shouldn't only be* my *decision.*

Cursing quietly, I slammed the car in park. *Had I read the signs wrong?*

David had said things like "If our family is complete right now, I am absolutely fine." While holding one of our atrociously spoiled cats, he would smile and comment, "I love everything about our little family." I thought I was reading between the lines.

But there were other signs that David wasn't okay with missing out on fatherhood.

Once when my parents were visiting, Mom and I were upstairs cleaning out my closet. Dad and David were downstairs in the basement. As she held up an old sweater ("keep or donate?"), we heard angry footsteps below.

Shortly after came a house-shaking slam of the front door, and finally, the sound of a car peeling out of the driveway. *What in the . . . ?*

David was gone for more than an hour, not returning my texts.

Later that evening, I learned the full story. David spoke in a strangled whisper, still obviously shaken.

"Your dad said, 'I hope you know that we respect your decision not to have kids. I would have loved to have been a grandfather, but that wouldn't have been fair to you. Or to us.'"

David exhaled. I closed my eyes.

No, Dad did not say that. Yet, of course he did. *Oh God.*

Never put it past Dad to say the exact wrong thing, in all of his love and sincerity.

<hr />

I slammed the car door in the parking garage. *That bloody tampon, though.* The thought brought me back to the present and propelled me forward, into the elevator at the gynecologist's office.

The receptionist asked for my name. I handed her my driver's license. Since I was already holding back tears, I knew she wouldn't understand my speech. Another doctor's office, another set of intake forms. I settled into a chair to fill out paperwork with infuriatingly slow handwriting.

"I don't understand why we have to go through genetic counseling again. Everything was fine with Liam," a man said to his visibly pregnant wife, gesturing at the toddler.

Liam, I presume. The toddler had been openly staring at me. He waddled toward me, arms outstretched. I smiled big to let him know that people with disabilities aren't scary.

The pregnant lady responded to the man, "Because the genes could have combined differently this time. It's better to be safe than sorry, and anyway—Liam! Get away from that lady's walker!"

Liam was attempting to push the walker, just like he'd seen me do. His mom jumped up, with surprising speed considering her protruding belly, and steered him away.

See? I thought for the umpteenth time. *I couldn't have done that.*

Whenever I was around children and parents, I played a twisted game in my mind: *What things could I not do as a parent?* I couldn't stop a kid from running into the street, putting their hand on a hot burner, or popping something dangerous into their mouth. And while I knew that disabled people could be incredible parents, my disease would eventually make every physical task impossible.

Hell, I couldn't even stop our cats from fighting.

In today's round of my twisted game: my kid would be making off with all the walkers in the room, including my own, and I couldn't do a damn thing to stop it.

"Andrea Peet?" The nurse called me back to the exam room.

As I pushed past Liam, I took one last look at him. He had climbed up on a chair much too high for him. The back legs of the chair lifted off the floor, and as I walked through the door, I heard "Liam, no!"

See? I couldn't have done that. No way can I be a mother.

The door closed firmly behind me.

CHAPTER 21

TRIALS

November 2015

If I was going to give myself a chance to live—even a (very) long-shot chance—I needed to get a move on and enroll in a clinical trial. My eligibility clock was ticking. Loudly.

Since the one ALS drug approved at the time only extended life by two or three months, my only other pharmaceutical avenue was to enroll in a clinical trial to try out an experimental drug. Most clinical trials only allow patients to enroll two to three years from their diagnosis date, including a diagnosis of probable ALS, which meant my eligibility clock started ticking in May 2014.

Why? Why would pharmaceutical companies exclude people with a terminal disease from trying to save their lives through a clinical trial after only two to three years?

Because if you're still alive after that point, they assume you have a slower progressing form of ALS. In other words, the researchers can't tell if their experimental drug is working . . . or if it's just *you*, and your unique brand of ALS.

I enrolled in the Phase III clinical trial of a drug to strengthen lung muscles, since respiratory failure is the actual cause of death for most people with ALS. Phase III meant that it was likely the last hurdle before FDA approval—assuming the drug worked.

Everything was fine on Monday when I started the treatment.

By Tuesday, I felt like I was trying to stay awake after taking a sleeping pill.

By Wednesday, I asked my acupuncturist to forgo the treatment she'd planned on my perpetually too-tight hamstrings in favor of an antivertigo treatment. Afterward, I curled up on the couch to minimize the world spinning.

By Thursday, I was even more groggy, dizzy, and sluggish. Even so, I went to lunch with a friend. She told me that Lisa's husband Sean was dating again. Lisa had just died six months ago.

I felt a shaking begin somewhere so deep inside I had no idea where it started. I knew Lisa wanted Sean to get married again and have kids, just like I wanted for David.

Eventually, yes. But so soon? I pushed the thought away. I closed my eyes, clasped my fingers together to stop the trembling, and leaned back in my chair.

Somehow, I got through lunch and back into my car. A light drizzle broke through the overcast day. I still shook but could at least grasp the steering wheel in the crawling DC traffic.

Apparently, a bomb scare had snarled traffic more than usual. I was grateful for the fogginess in my head from the clinical trial drug. It muted all thoughts. Well, except this one: *How could he be dating already?*

I walked into the house and flung myself on the couch. I cried until I fell asleep. When I woke up, the house was dark and quiet. I had slept for more than three hours.

I called David's work number. No answer. His cell. No answer. I sent a text. No response. I fed the cats. I had a snack. I did some laundry and packed for our trip to Boston the next day. But my phone sat on the bed, silent.

By 9 P.M., I had run out of things to do and David had still not called. My body shaking was back. *There's no explanation for this! He never misses a call, and when he does, he returns it quickly—especially if there are six missed calls.*

My mind—in all its fogginess—went straight there. *He must be having an affair.*

That thought had such a hold on me that I couldn't walk, so I curled up on the bed and just tormented myself with the vision: David making passionate love to some faceless woman. It must be a coworker. I pictured them in his office, on his desk. She was straddling him with her legs wrapped around his back in ways I could no longer do.

Before I could sink any lower, I heard the front door click open.

"Hello?" David called out.

He walked into the bedroom, saw my face, and said, "Oh, babe! What's wrong?"

Sinking down next to me on the bed, he pulled me into his arms. I buried my face in his chest, sobbing and sputtering into his blue button-down shirt. He let me cry for a long while, stroking my hair.

When I pulled myself together enough to choke out the news about Sean having a new girlfriend, he seemed genuinely shocked, which comforted me.

"Oh, babe," he said.

"And then, when I couldn't reach you, I thought . . ." I couldn't finish my sentence.

"Oh, babe," he said again. "I was stuck in the Metro. There was a broken train. A bomb scare caused all sorts of issues."

Of course. The Metro: the one place cell service goes to die. My beautiful, wonderful, honorable husband. I would have felt ridiculous if I hadn't been so miserable.*

⌘

By 10 A.M. the next morning, I was in a conference room of a Boston hotel fully submerged in the heavy science of ALS, not absorbing any of it. David had gone to his firm's Boston office to work for the day while I sat in lectures.

I was attending the ALS Therapy Development Institute (ALS TDI) conference. ALS TDI is a nonprofit research lab in Watertown, Massachusetts. Our Team Drea funds continually support their research, and I am an "ambassador" for their Young Faces of ALS campaign.

The lecture might have been over my head even if I was not fighting the foggy side effects of a trial drug. A researcher from ALS TDI shared the latest

---

* Later, I heard from other friends that they had strange hallucinations or paranoias from the trial drug. One friend deleted all of his social media, convinced he was being spied on.

findings, a slide that showed three MRI scans of a mouse taken at two-hour intervals. I was so out of it all I could think was: *How do you get a mouse to sit still enough for an MRI?* Things were getting weirder by the minute.

During the break, I stood up and immediately sat back down. The room was spinning. I tried again to take some steps forward, but my toes dragged. I could not overpower my foot drop. David wasn't there; no one was. I was too unsteady to cross the room by myself, even with my walker.

I called the clinical trial coordinator and, through slurred words, managed to ask her what I should do.

"How do I know when the side effects are too much? I don't want to hurt the trial by dropping out, but I feel awful."

"It's up to you," she said sympathetically—which was true, and also completely unhelpful.

I was in the hotel bed by 6 P.M. I woke up just long enough to eat the takeout David brought me. We watched news coverage of terrorist attacks in Paris, gunmen and suicide bombers from the Islamic State assaulting a concert hall, a stadium, and popular nightlife spots. I wondered if I was hallucinating again. *Has the whole world gone crazy?*

At 4 A.M., I woke up with the clearest single thought I'd had all week: *I've had enough. I'm out. I can't control much about this disease and I may die more quickly without this drug, but I will not live my life this way.*

The clinical trial drug ultimately failed to slow the decline of lung capacity in patients with ALS. Hundreds of patients and millions of dollars later? Back to the drawing board.

CHAPTER 22

HOME SWEET HOME

January 2016

"What is your heart telling you?" David asked me as we tag-teamed the nightly dishes.

I stopped, mid-rinse on a glass, and looked at him. David did not normally talk that way.

My bottom lip quivered. I handed him the glass and turned back to the sink. *Keep it together, Drea.*

"Hey," he said quietly. "What is it?"

I turned, leaned in, and buried my face in David's flannel shirt.

"It's okay, love. You don't have to know right now," he said.

I was crying. Hard. Not because I didn't know. Rather, I was crying because I *did*.

"I want to go *home*," I sobbed.

He knew what I meant. *Home.* We were standing in our kitchen in Maryland, but I wanted to go *home*-home. Home to North Carolina. Home to my parents. That's the thing about dying. Suddenly, priorities become really clear. The courage to voice those priorities? Well, that sometimes takes longer.

The problem forcing the issue was our house.

A ginormous ALS wheelchair wouldn't fit in the bathroom, down the hall, or through the doorway of our 1960s-era house. The contractor made the list look easy. He would relocate a few walls here, move a closet there, redo the bathroom plumbing—*voilà!* But when I saw the number of zeroes involved in *voilà!*, I nearly threw the computer across the room.

Question: How does anyone with ALS afford this?

Answer: Most can't.

ALS groups were filled with sad stories of draining retirement savings for home renovations. Some asked for advice on bankruptcy or entering hospice to qualify for nursing assistance at home. One couple got divorced so the spouse with ALS could enroll in Medicaid while the other spouse used their savings to renovate. Those who could not afford to move or renovate tended to spend their final days in a living room or dining room, peeing in a bedpan.

While we were exceedingly fortunate to be able to afford renovations, considering such a massive investment made me assess the big picture realistically. My world had started shrinking again.

I didn't feel safe on the Metro, so I resorted to driving. Driving meant parking. Parking meant circling the block multiple times to find a space close enough to access with my walker. I learned which parking garages validated with purchase, which had excellent handicapped-accessible parking spaces, and which were downright scary.

In graduate school, my master's project was to create a downtown parking plan for a small town in the Atlanta suburbs. I drew maps. I spent days walking the downtown area, counting thousands of parking spaces. I studied parking patterns. With all my naïve grad student bravado, I recommended policies about shared parking, street parking, and fees. Never once did I address *accessible* parking for people with mobility issues.

In other words, I was now being served with straight-up parking karma.

While certain that my current parking woes were punishment from the parking gods, I reminded myself how lucky I was. I could still drive. We could afford a car and exorbitant parking fees. But even in gratitude, I had lost access to the things I loved about my city. I was staying home more. Everything would continue to grow in difficulty as ALS progressed.

More than anything, I wanted to reconnect with my parents. Not for them to take care of me, but to repair our relationship. I was their only child after all, and they were getting older. I missed them. And before I died, I wanted to make sure they knew how much I loved them.

I cried in the kitchen because, as hard as my situation was, I knew what I was asking of David.

After all the stressful years and hours paying his dues at the big DC law firm, he would be cutting his legal career short because of me. He would not make partner working remotely—if it was even an option to keep his job.

Worse still, with this one request, I was asking him to give up *his* family in favor of *mine*.

Washington, DC, had been a perfect spot, geographically centered between our parents. His sister and her family lived close enough to hang out almost every weekend. And since I had foreclosed the possibility of kids for us, David had poured his dad-like love into his niece and nephew.

I cried because of what I was asking. But I also cried because I knew he would say yes. Which of course he did.

As I always told people, "I swear, I knew he was the best man when I married him, but I had no idea."

I bargained with myself. *It's only for a couple of years. Once I'm gone, he can move back up here and pick up his life again.*

⬥

Two months later, the movers dumped our stuff into our first-floor, ADA-accessible apartment in Raleigh. As soon as they left, I made a beeline for the nearby Lifetime Fitness mega-gym and joined. Forget the multiple pools and towel service, let's talk about the twenty accessible parking spaces right out front—now *that* was downright luxurious. I almost cried at the automatic door that opened with just the push of a button. *Have the parking gods forgiven me?*

My parents and I established a routine of doing what we did best: *work*. Twice a week, while Dad joined the other retirees kicking and grooving to the music of aqua aerobics, Mom and I got busy in the shallow end of the pool. We built a workout routine of squats, lunges, stretches of all types. Mom bought new equipment to try: a noodle, swim fins, a push plate, and resistance hand paddles that resembled enormous crab claws.

I was at once horrified by all that I could—and could *not*—do.

Each session, I practiced walking the length of the pool, my hands gripping a noodle for balance, reminding my body of this process that used to come naturally. The walking exercises reminded me of learning Spanish while studying abroad. While my friends seemed to converse easily with native speakers, I never graduated past the clunky process of translating each word and conjugating verbs. Now at Lifetime, I was conjugating walking, piece by piece. *Shift your weight, foot up, toes up, pass it through . . .*

I tried swimming. I could pull myself through the water with my arms, gasping for breath. I could make it to the other side, but it was a challenge. I could not kick—like, at all.

Mom walked behind me. That way, she could yank her baby out of the water at the first sign of trouble.

But the hardest exercise of all was keeping my mouth shut.

I kept my jaw tight to prevent the words in my brain from escaping into the air. I loved the *idea* of being with my parents. The *reality* of being with my parents often left me seething inside. Their constant hovering and loving vigilance made me feel like a toddler. Their actions were a well-intentioned series of desperate attempts to keep their little girl from struggling.

Dad insisted on meeting me in the parking lot each day to "help" me into the gym. I reminded him of the automatic door opener. He waved me off. Mom constantly reached for my bag to take it from me.

"I can do it myself!" I hissed (all the time). I immediately felt guilty (all the time).

Of course, Andy and Sandy were just so happy I was home again. I knew that. *What kind of a daughter gets angry at her parents for over-helping, over-doing, over-loving?*

But *I* wanted to do all the things, for myself. To prove to my parents that I was still able. To prove to myself. To preserve a few remaining shreds of independence before ALS took it away. *You'll be back to having to wipe my butt soon enough, Mom and Dad. Just be patient.*

I was mad at my parents for not recognizing what I needed (or didn't need). I was madder at myself for my impatience. When I felt overly parented, I regressed to a bratty teenager or, worse, a bratty two-year-old. I felt awful. We hadn't moved back for me to tear apart our relationship further. We moved home so I could rebuild it. I was doing a terrible job. And I made sure to beat myself up for it daily.

I wanted to stop the circle of guilt—where speaking my mind led to hurting their feelings, then feeling guilty for hurting them even though I was just trying to establish what I needed (and didn't), and on and on. A vicious cycle that I had no idea how to break out of.

A bigger problem: I recognized how much older they had become. Now in their mid-seventies, they moved slower, ate slower, processed thoughts slower. It scared me. So, I covered over my sadness and fear with impatience.

Especially because they couldn't understand me.

David had learned my speech patterns. My friends only asked me to repeat things occasionally. But my parents responded to nearly everything with "huh?"

Dad had needed hearing aids for years—long before my speech went downhill. He refused. Just like he resisted getting a cane, or a smartphone, or anything else he refused for whatever reason. So I often raised my voice (in both volume and frustration). He still couldn't understand me.

"Sorry," he said, "I'm just not getting it." My face burned with anger, and then I reverted to either sixteen- or two-year-old Andrea, depending on the day. *Why are you so mean, Andrea?*

Eventually, I filtered what I chose to say. *Is this really a story worth the frustration of repeating?* I'd calculate in my head. Usually, no. During our conversations, I kept quiet. I let Dad ramble on about anything he wanted to discuss, which was usually lawn mowing related.

I adopted a new policy with myself: you can say absolutely anything inside your head, but what comes out of your mouth must be kind.

When Mom hovered as I got on the ladder in the pool, my brain would say: *OMG, stop hovering. Have I ever fallen off the ladder? Have I ever even stumbled?*

But what came out was a calm, but assertive, "I'm fine. You can go get the noodles if you want to."

With my assertion, she got the hint. I was freed from my guilt.

Was there a crack in the guilt circle?

CHAPTER 23

TATTOOS

May 2016

I got a tattoo. Me, the eager-to-please only child? Me, the didn't-drink-till-I-was-21 rule follower? Me, the super goody-goody? Yep, I got a tattoo. *I am a fucking rebel.*

Like everyone with ALS, one grim statistic had haunted me since the day I was diagnosed: *the average life expectancy is two to five years.* Like everyone with ALS, that knowledge pressed down on my heart, seeped into my bones. Impossible to avoid, extinguishing all possibility of Hope.

Impossible, too, to know the pace of progression. Only time would tell—the cruelest statistic of all.

Most neurologists regard the pace of progression as linear.

By that measure, I figured I was screwed.

Only six months passed between the time I finished the half-distance triathlon and when I found myself lying in the street unable to get up. Jon Blais lived two years. Jillaine and Jodi's mom lived fourteen months. Lisa lived thirteen months.

So, two years after my probable ALS diagnosis, I got a tattoo. Two years felt like a giant milestone. Maybe, rather, a deep breath slowly exhaled. A breath I didn't realize I was holding.

My friend with ALS Arthur Cohen said, "Until further notice, celebrate everything." I felt like celebrating.

In *Big Magic*, Elizabeth Gilbert writes about a friend who "acquires new tattoos the way I might buy a new pair of earrings." Her friend explained, "My tattoos are permanent. It's my *body* that's temporary. . . . We're here on earth for a very short while. I just want to decorate my temporary self as playfully and beautifully as I can, while I still have time."

Considering how short my stay would be, I wanted to get on with this decorating business. And I knew *exactly* which tattoo to get.

In 2009 and a few towns away, a twenty-nine-year-old named Tim LaFollette* began experiencing foot drop. While I was stressing myself out over wedding planning, Tim received his ALS diagnosis. He had hoped a recent bike accident caused the symptoms, but the doctors were suspicious, due to Tim's family history.

In 1982, his mother died of ALS, and months later, his grandmother. At the time, the genetic form of ALS was unknown, so the string of events was assumed to be a series of unlucky coincidences. But Tim's family identified symptoms in at least five generations—dating back to 1903—twenty-seven years before Lou Gehrig's famous speech.

Tim tattooed the swallows from his mother's Quaker songbook on his arm—a whole flock of black birds in flight.

In traditional tattoo lore, swallows are a symbol of Hope. Sailors tattooed swallows on their bodies because when swallows appeared at sea, they signaled nearby land—the sailor knew he was almost home. Many others in Tim's circle began to ink swallow tattoos in solidarity. They called themselves the Often Awesome Army, and they stayed by Tim's side until he died in 2011.

My current neurologist (and Tim's doctor), Dr. Rick Bedlack at Duke, has a small swallow on his hand. He said, "When I sign a patient's chart, my tattoo pops out of my sleeve. It reminds me to tell my patient something hopeful."

A Doctor of Hope—in ALS. Now *that* is unusual, but so is Dr. Bedlack. His appearance outwardly screams it—and he saves his best outfits for his patients. He might show up to the ALS Clinic in a fabulous toile-print suit, completed with plastic Buddy Holly glasses and spiked hair. He understands

---

* Tim and his partner, Kaylan, chronicled their journey with his disease in short documentaries called *Often Awesome: The Series*.

that ALS is a tough disease for his patients, so some dapper clothes might bring a smile or two.

Dr. Bedlack embraces the ethos of Fox Mulder from the *X-Files*, the UFO show whose poster proclaims "I WANT TO BELIEVE." Dr. Bedlack believes in Hope and is willing to think outside the box to help his patients. For example, through the ALS Untangled program, Dr. Bedlack and his merry band of neurological volunteers study the science behind nutritional supplements that some living with ALS swear have helped their symptoms.

He has also begun studying the alien-equivalent in ALS: *reversals*. Actual people with actual documented cases of ALS whose symptoms reversed course, allowing them to go on to enjoy full, healthy lives. He has found almost sixty—out of 30,000 living in the US at any one time. But, still, they exist. There is Hope.

I had spent the last two years trying to wrap my brain around how to live a life when there's no Hope. But Dr. Bedlack lives with Hope; he built his career on it. Hope drives his quest to find a cure. I want to believe he will.

For my tattoo, I wanted two swallows for two years. Two swallows for two marathons. Two swallows for David and me.

At first, I wanted to put them somewhere subtle, somewhere I could cover up. But what was I worried about, not looking professional? Someone not hiring me?

"You're not serious," Mom said when I told her. "I always checked you for tattoos when you came home from college, remember?"

"Why would you get a tattoo?" Dad asked.

Well, that sealed my decision. I would be the rebellious teenager in my thirties that I never was in my teens. The swallow pair would perch right on my forearm where everyone could see them—especially me.

In late May, I pushed my walker through the doors of a tattoo shop with David and Julie in tow. With the needle pounding my skin, I had an idea. *I will get one new swallow every May, to celebrate the milestone of making it one more year. One more year of Hope.*

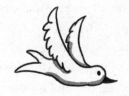

CHAPTER 24

FLYING ON ONE ENGINE

January 2017

I kept swimming, kept trying with my parents, twice a week, every week. My muscles grew stronger, and they weren't ridiculously tight any longer. My patience grew, too.

"Your body is always trying to heal itself," Mom would say. She always said this. Followed by—"I just wish you could find a PT down here." *Yep, there it is.*

In an online ALS group, I read about a woman with ALS working with a Pilates-based physical therapist. My friend Corey had mentioned Pilates too. He had been diagnosed at age twenty-one and swore that Pilates stretched his tight muscles. Considering he had been living with ALS for more than a decade, I listened.

So when Mom once again mentioned PT, I was prepared.

"Oh, I've been looking into Pilates-based PT," I said in my newly calm—but still know-it-all—voice.

"What's that?" she asked, which gave me the opportunity to smugly deliver my newly acquired knowledge. Which was precisely how Mom and I ended up at InsideOut Body Therapies in Durham, North Carolina.

"Did you know that Joseph Pilates actually developed his practice for bed-ridden patients?" Mischa Decker, the studio owner, told us.

"I didn't know Pilates was a person," I said.

Joseph Pilates was a German citizen detained in a British internment camp during World War I. While working as a hospital orderly, he rigged up bed springs for patients who were unable to walk.

"The springs offered the gentle resistance of the person's body weight, which helped them gradually build up strength," Mischa said.

Over the following months, she introduced me to the weird-looking spring machines with even weirder names: the Reformer, the Cadillac, the Core-Align. The machines forced me to pay attention to muscle groups that had weakened without me even noticing. Like my glutes.

"Your quads are so strong from triking—they are dominating everything else."

So, she took them out of the equation. She helped me down onto my back on the Cadillac. Nope, not the car—a Pilates machine that looks like a table attached to a metal frame resembling a canopy bed. Once secured, Mischa lifted my legs in springs attached to the vertical poles.

"Now try to scissor your legs."

I tried. Nothing happened. I squinted at my legs. *Yep, nope. Nothing.* I was trying, but no-go.

Mischa tapped the side of my right glute to cue which muscle to activate. *Okay, go!* When I concentrated with *all* my might, I felt my glutes and hamstrings engage to power my right leg downward.

Mischa began counting. "Let's try for five. One . . ."

And such began the torment that was Pilates. My legs barely moved. It looked like nothing. But I was sweating.

"Does that feel like work?" Mischa asked.

I cracked up at her ridiculous question. Then I couldn't stop laughing. My giggles infected Mischa—and we traded laughs for a while. Mom (always present at my appointments) looked confused, but even she chuckled.

Mischa was a game changer. Her cues, telling my muscles to individually activate, were a literal turning point. Mentally, I pictured the motor neurons stretching down from my brain and spinal cortex to the intended muscles. *Flex, flex, flex.* And miracles of miracles, my muscles responded. All slow, some with extreme concentration, but if I could move them, then the *connection* to the muscle wasn't dead. And that meant *everything.* That meant *life.*

Through sessions with Mischa, I learned the map of my body. I felt the chains of muscles supporting my hips, thighs, knees, ankles, even my big toes. These chains of fibers propelled me forward in the ingenious concept of *walking.*

While my muscles had forgotten what to do on their own, if I concentrated hard enough, my mind could cue the muscles. Then my mind could order them to cooperate.

Pilates gave my pool workouts new meaning and purpose, and some clarity for my sessions with Mom. We both felt the excitement of progress.

I walked back and forth along the black line at the bottom of the pool, my gaze fixed on the middle distance of the horizon, concentrating so hard my mouth would fall open. One excruciatingly slow lap after another, I navigated the map of my muscles. *Shift your weight, foot up, toes up, pass it through, tense your core to maintain balance, land with the heel, roll through the foot. Yes! Shift your weight. Again. Go.*

"Great job!" Mom would say after a particularly good lap. "You know, your body is always trying to heal itself."

"I know," I said, giving her the tiniest smile. But a real one. *She's not wrong.*

❧

In March 2017, an *ALS News Today* article caught my eye: "Could Exercise Help ALS Patients with Swallowing?" To date, anything encouraging exercise in ALS was pretty much taboo. Not even Dr. Bedlack put much stock in it—he just thought I was an outlier with extraordinarily slow progression.

The lead researcher, Dr. Emily Plowman at the University of Florida, worked as a speech language pathologist in an ALS Clinic. She was frustrated. In her role, she could only offer ALS patients feeding tubes or technological solutions for their voices, like text-to-speech apps or eye-gaze computers—but that was it. No help, no therapies.

"Historically, exercise has been sort of 'boo-hooed' in this patient population, that it would hasten patient progression. However, this is unfounded. There's no big empirical evidence to support this statement," Dr. Plowman said in the video posted with the article. *Wait, what?*

She went on to say that research on other neurological diseases, such as Parkinson's and Muscular dystrophy, showed that exercise was beneficial for patients. A small study with ALS mice revealed exercise as "neuroprotective," thus increasing survival rates.

Well, hello, lovely! A researcher after Mom's own heart. At each visit to the ALS Clinic, I'd find Mom in the waiting room reading the Parkinson's bulletin board.

"Look at this!" she'd exclaim. "They have *kickboxing* for Parkinson's patients!" Or yoga. Or dancing. Inwardly, I'd roll my eyes, knowing what was coming.

"When will ALS get it together?" *There it is.*

"But they are different diseases," I'd always respond, not knowing why I was defending the glacial pace of ALS research. My default reflex to be adversarial felt especially teenage-y on this point. *Wasn't I living proof that exercise was beneficial?*

Dr. Plowman's study tested respiratory muscle training—essentially weight training for the lungs and diaphragm. She asked the question: Could exercising those muscles improve swallowing and breathing?

I was captivated. What would all my success strengthening my muscles through Pilates, swimming, and triking mean if I could no longer breathe? Nothing—I'd be dead.

I wrote Dr. Plowman to ask if I could participate.

Dr. Plowman wrote back: "I accept anyone who is willing to come to Gainesville, Florida, twice"—once at the beginning of the three-month study, and once at the end. The check-in sessions would be by video chat.

Mom and I bought plane tickets to Florida that day.

⌘

Dr. Plowman handed me an expiratory muscle strength trainer. Slightly bigger than a tube of toothpaste with a mouthpiece at one end, the device had a coiled spring inside with a dial to ratchet up the tension. After the nose plugs were in place, she instructed me to take a deep breath and exhale as hard and fast as I could into the device.

"There," Dr. Plowman said. "That's one rep."

She found my "maximum expiratory pressure" (the point at which it was too difficult for me to blow), calculated 30 percent of that, and set the spirometer accordingly.

We repeated the process with an inspiratory device for inhaling.

"You'll use each device—both inhale and exhale—five days a week." She spouted off reps and timing in the same manner as weight training.

The plan was to check in every other week via video call. My goal was to increase the "weight" by increasing the tension on the springs. *A goal! I like.*

"The best part?" Dr. Plowman continued. "These trainers are available online for about fifty bucks each."

I was floored. *That's it? One hundred bucks?*

The current choice for those living with ALS when respiratory function starts to fail is usually "non-invasive ventilation" (NIV) machines. More commonly called a bipap or Trilogy, the machine requires the person to be hooked up to a machine pumping air into their lungs through a plastic mask covering the nose and sometimes the mouth. Truly not a great way to live.

If Dr. Plowman's hypothesis was correct, people living with ALS could strengthen or maintain their respiratory system. Which might postpone needing a machine to help them breathe.

What if this simple set of exercises could delay the difficult decision to use a trach? What if the device sitting in my hand could give people more quality time with their families and loved ones?

And for only a hundred bucks.

⬥

After a long (but hopeful) day in Florida, Mom and I boarded our connecting flight in Atlanta at 10:30 P.M.

I had just begun to snooze after takeoff, when suddenly: *BOOM!* The plane lurched.

My eyes flew open to see sparks streaming past the window. I was in the middle seat, but the teenage girl in the window seat reported smoke coming from the wing, which we then smelled in the cabin. *Holy . . .*

After the explosion, the plane slowed but stayed level. *Comforting.*

Not so comforting, however, was the flight attendant pacing up and down the aisle shrieking, "Everyone stay calm!" This was a real emergency. And we all knew it.

Except for a few nervous whispers, a palpable hush fell over us—two hundred passengers. We were all holding our collective breath.

Mom was in the aisle seat next to me.

I reached for her hand and held it. We looked out the window. There was nothing else to do. I considered calling David. We were flying low enough for a cell signal. But what would I say to him? Goodbye? That we were going to crash? After everything we'd been through, I could not believe our story might end this way.

A phone call would have broken the silence on the plane. I didn't want to do that. The silence was just too powerful.

So I sat, holding Mom's hand, contemplating the reality that we might actually be about to die. How strange, to be on a crashing airplane, after being so certain that it was ALS that was going to get me. Talk about a plot twist.

In that moment, I experienced clarity, even peace, like never before.

I had been given the gift of time, which most people with ALS don't get. And I had an up-close perspective of how quickly time could be taken away. I had lived an amazing life with so much love, support, and magic around me. I was also impatient. And way too hard on myself. My relationship with my parents had been a work in progress.

But there Mom and I were. After all the ups and downs, we were holding hands, on a silent, perhaps crashing, plane. In that moment, I wanted to be with her. After all, I came into the world from her. She had given me so much. She had raised me to be strong and independent—and through it all, had stuck with me.

She never lost Hope. She had made it her mission to make me believe in Hope too. I exhaled.

I truly loved the company I was in.

After five long minutes, the captain announced that the left engine was blown. He continued, "We can fly with one engine; we do it all the time.* The bad news is that we're heading back to Atlanta."

The next half hour involved a series of slow loops as we descended. The slow, circular motion gave all passengers ample time and metaphor to ponder the meaning of life, the universe—you know, the usual.

Had this been my first rodeo with death, I might have reacted like the twentysomething woman in front of us, shaking and sobbing uncontrollably. Maybe I would have made all sorts of promises to get my life in order. Focus on the big picture. Do all the things I had been putting off.

But I had been actively mining those questions and answers and plans and promises for three years. I needed no more time for that.

Instead, I simply held Mom's hand, breathed deeply, and was grateful for the opportunity to do just that. We eventually landed in Atlanta. We held hands a little longer, even as we rolled up to the gate.

The truth is, we're all flying on one engine . . . whether we realize it or not.

---

* This line turned out to be a massive overstatement. Another flight attendant told us later that in her twenty-year career, she'd never been on a plane that blew out an engine. *Go figure.*

PART III

HOPE
FIGHTS
BACK

CHAPTER 25

GET IT ON FILM

February–April 2019

By 2019, life was good. I was alive and had a solid routine. I swam twice a week, saw Mischa at Pilates once a week, and triked on weekends. I had finished twelve races each year since 2016—of all different distances. We moved into our accessible, one-floor forever home (after a huge renovation—more on that later). David had a new partner-track job at a local law firm.

While I wasn't one of Dr. Bedlack's miraculous ALS reversals, I was clearly not in danger of imminent death either.

I maintained a constant vigilance: *concentrate while speaking; exercise to stave off weakness and tight muscles.* I could still drive, talk, eat, dress myself, get around with a walker, and run the daily operations of the Team Drea Foundation.

As appreciative as I was, I had to admit that I was getting a little bored. It's weird when you end up living longer than you expected—eventually the monotony of everyday life creeps back in.

"Have you ever thought about having someone film a documentary about your journey?" Keith asked.

Keith was a sports marketing consultant. My friend Shaw and I were on a call with him, hoping to spark some sponsor interest in my story. Keith gently let us know how unlikely that was, given that I was an amateur nobody, ALS or not.

In a last-ditch effort to keep the conversation going, I unleashed my crazy idea on Keith. The one I had been toying around with for several months.

"What if . . . I completed a marathon in every state?" I asked.

I had finished marathons in six states. So, a "mere" forty-four more to go.

The fifty-in-fifty idea snagged his attention, and Keith liked the concept. I liked it because it was a challenge and different from my day-to-day life. A goal. *Okay, fifty marathons is out in the open now.*

But a documentary? That had never crossed my mind.

⤙⤚

In January, I'd visited my college roommate, Elizabeth, in South Carolina. Since I was visiting anyway, why not bring the trike and do the Charleston Marathon? *Sounded like a plan to me!*

During the race, as I pedaled past the Southern mansions along the Battery, I realized how much I still loved exploring new cities. And marathons would be a great way to do that. After all, streets were closed to cars during a marathon. My inner urban-planner-geek could (safely) gawk at local architecture and explore neighborhoods from the center of the road.

Marathons, however, also give you a lot of time to think. Maybe too much time.

I wondered how many marathons I could finish before ALS caught up with me. Could I finish one in every state? Since 2016, I had ticked off four states: North Carolina (#1), Virginia (#2), Ohio (#3), and now South Carolina (#4). That's where the fifty-in-fifty idea started to brew.

Plus, my fifth anniversary with ALS was approaching. Considering that only 20 percent of people lived past five years with ALS, the milestone felt monumental.

My friend Eddy tattooed his fifth ALS anniversary date on his arm. His "expiration date," he called it. The tattoo literally read "EXP. 04/97," like a carton of milk. And yet, he lived twenty-one more years with ALS *after* that date.

With my expiration date approaching, I was still completing marathons. I shook my helmeted head in disbelief. Never, ever could I have predicted I'd still be alive—let alone racing. Not with how fast my early progression had been.

Could I be like Eddy and live for decades?

Until recently, I had refused to let that question even slip into my thoughts. *Could I actually live?* After my diagnosis, I had scrubbed and bleached all future plans and dreams from my mind. I had wrung them out, folded them up neatly, and put them away in an imaginary drawer inside of myself.

Did I dare open it again?

Darcy Wakefield, in her memoir *I Remember Running*, wrote that she woke up every morning and checked if her ALS had reversed. It hadn't, and she died two years later.

I had taken the opposite approach. I worked daily to accept that I would die; it was my badge of pragmatism. *Stop contributing to your 401(k). Do one last triathlon before your body fails you. Don't have kids. Stay ahead of the disease. Write your will. Get a blender that will liquefy chili.*

I had organized the shit out of the life I had left.

But *what if* the magic reversal was *not* an overnight miracle like Darcy hoped for? What if the magic was a mere sliver of a chance for reversal before the nerve connections to the muscles flamed out for good? Maybe all the triking and swimming and Pilates and respiratory muscle training had held my brain-nerve-muscle connections intact. *What if . . .*

If the journey of a thousand miles cliché begins with a single step, perhaps I'd already been on the path for a while. *Fifty marathons*. I loved the idea. I loved the Hope of fifty marathons.

⚯

"What do you want to do for your birthday?" David asked.

"A race. Duh," I said, smiling. "Maybe in Austin."

Of course, I'd already researched the marathons on my February birthday weekend. Then, I took a breath and told him my crazy idea about a marathon in all fifty states. (Right, I hadn't told David yet. I know, I know—poor David.)

There was a pause.

"Well, okay then," David said. "If that's what you really want to do." Because of course he would say that.

The journey of a thousand miles had, in fact, already begun. A journey of 1,310 miles, to be exact: fifty marathons, in fifty different states, 26.2 miles each.

Texas, Georgia, and Tennessee: Marathons #5, #6, and #7 February–April 2019

We woke up at 2:30 A.M. to catch an early flight to Texas (#5).

David and I had perfected flying with the trike. Airlines didn't bat an eye when we presented the trike as a "mobility device." It was checked for free as oversized baggage.

Protecting the trike from damage was a different story. Dad helped me pack the trike. The former drafting teacher grinned with gleeful pride—the only thing he loved more than a challenge and lawn mowing was helping his daughter.

His methodology was a work of art. Dad carefully pulled golf club putter covers over each pedal. He delicately encased the trike's critical components (shifters, derailleur, gears) in bubble wrap while I hobbled around on my walker, handing him strips of packing tape. I then stuffed our suitcase with an equivalent amount of bubble wrap, tape, and scissors for David to rewrap everything for the return flight.

The trike looked like the Michelin Man—all bubbled and floaty-like. No box, just a floating cloud of bubbles. Finally, we labeled the floating cloud: "WHEELCHAIR: DO NOT TURN UPSIDE DOWN!"

Dad did this for me before every race. A simple, supportive gesture from him. Chief Trike Wrapper.

David and I touched down in Austin. I watched from my window seat as the baggage handlers unloaded the plane. Sure enough, a bubble-wrapped *upside-down* trike came down the conveyor belt. *Dammit.*

We inspected the trike in baggage claim. And sure enough, torn bubble wrap revealed a broken shifter. *Dammit.* As much as I wanted to make a bee-line to the nearest bike shop, I could tell David was exhausted from our early morning. Me too. Coffee first.

Sufficiently caffeinated, we found a bike shop and fortunately, the shifter was easily repaired.

We got lucky. I feared that wouldn't always be the case.

⤫

Later that night, David and I dined by candlelight in the hotel restaurant. Knowing it was a luxury many of my friends with ALS could no longer enjoy, I soaked it in. We laughed, really talked, and were in bed by 8:30 P.M.

On race morning, we joined 17,000 runners walking toward the start line of the Austin Marathon. We made our way to the front, where the only other "wheeler" introduced herself from her seat in a handcycle.

"How many marathons have you done?" I asked.

"This will be my eighty-ninth marathon," she said. David and I both stared at her. *Wow.*

Beth Sanden had been partially paralyzed in a bicycle accident. She regained some mobility and was able to walk with a cane. She finished marathons on all seven continents, including Antarctica, where it was fifty below—and lost some fingernails. I later learned she had completed seven marathons in seven African countries in eight days, ending on her sixty-third birthday. Maybe doing fifty marathons wasn't so crazy, after all.

The race started. Beth disappeared out of sight within a few minutes—an immediate reminder of how different our conditions and our adaptive vehicles were. I moved to the right as the fastest runners passed. I settled into the rhythm of thudding feet all around me. Since diagnosis, I chose not to wear headphones or a watch during races. I wanted to hear the cheers and stay present in the experience. But that meant I was never sure of my speed until I spotted a pace group.

Pace groups are usually led by a volunteer runner who carries a large sign on a stick with a finish time posted. Runners who join up with the group can expect to finish around the time on the sign. This helps runners stay on top of their goal without obsessing over or fussing with their pace, and feel the camaraderie of a group with a similar goal.

As the race reached a steep downhill, I began flying past pace groups. I caught up to the 3:05 group, which made me so giddy and giggly that I started waving like a maniac to all the volunteers and spectators. My PR (personal record) was 3:34. *How crazy!*

I had been thinking about the Boston Marathon. If I were to *run* that sacred marathon, the qualifying time for my age group and gender would be 3:35. I wondered if Boston would let me in on my trike with that time. I'd already learned that a recumbent trike was not a "standard" adaptive vehicle. *But surely if I made it all the way to fifty marathons—with ALS—they'd make an exception . . .*

At mile 8, the race route turned a corner and ran smack into a hill. Like a holy-moly-what-the-hell-do-I-do monster of a hill. Gripping my brakes so I wouldn't roll backward, I paused to consider my options. *Should I ask someone to push me?* I doubted anyone could understand me. My breathless voice would be worse than usual. I tried to make eye contact with someone walking past me. No one was even pretending to run, the hill was so steep.

Panic set in. Not since my first marathon at City of Oaks had I encountered a hill this steep. David had pushed me up, while Julie walked alongside. Now I had no one.

I took a deep breath, eased off the brake, and started pushing down on the pedal with all my might. Only half a rotation, but the trike moved forward—at least a few inches. *Got it. This is how I do it.*

I backpedaled to give my right leg maximum leverage. Half rotation. Clamp on brakes. Backpedal. Switch legs. Again.

That's the way I made it up the monstrous hill and three more just like it.

The 3:05 group was long gone. I was hanging out with the 3:30 pacer and his flock. *But that will still give me a PR . . .*

At mile 26—a mere 0.2 miles from the end—another doozy of a hill. My heart sank. I had no power left in my legs, and I felt my new PR slipping away.

Suddenly, David appeared.

"You got this, you got this!" he shouted. And then to the crowd, "Make some noise!" All the spectators began cheering. With a smile on my face, I started cranking. At the top of the hill, I took off to the finish line.

3:32. PR! Yes!

❧

The Publix Atlanta Marathon (#6) was a few weeks later.

I lined up with wheeled athletes and push teams from the Kyle Pease Foundation.[1] Never before had I started with so many other wheelers, many of whom had cerebral palsy or other cognitive and physical limitations.

At the start line, everyone talked excitedly, fist-bumped, hugged, and prepared for the journey ahead. When the race started, a huge cheer rose up from spectators lining the course. The participants smiled and waved. *Where else does this happen in real life?* I thought, grinning and waving myself. *There is just nothing like a marathon—especially one that allows everyone to participate.*

Inclusion is essential to Atlanta Track Club's mission in all their events.

"We do whatever is in our power to make an accommodation for racers who want to participate," said Jay Holder, vice president of marketing and communications at the Atlanta Track Club said. "People seek out running events because of the way participating makes them feel. So we care deeply about inclusion [and] that is why I come to work every day."

"We have partnered with the Kyle Pease Foundation (push-assist athletes) for years, and we take pride in making sure that the local Atlanta and national running community is represented at this event, which is truly for everyone."

Inclusion. What a beautiful thing.

❧

The documentary idea—from the call with the sports consultant, Keith—hadn't gone anywhere, since I had no clue how to make a movie. That is, until two weeks after Atlanta.

When the local public broadcasting station sent a film crew to do a story about me, I found myself making small talk with a local videographer named Miriam—MJ for short. Her husband, Brian, ran a nonprofit organization for orphaned and at-risk youth in Rwanda. The stories MJ and Brian told through short films helped raise money for their nonprofit to help the youth in Africa.

The stars had aligned.

With no budget and no plan, MJ and Brian started shooting a documentary trailer about my dream to do fifty marathons.

This feels reckless, crazy, I thought as I caught sight of MJ and David running down a hill toward me in Nashville at the Rock 'n' Roll Marathon (#7).

Five years into ALS and now *I'm taking on fifty marathons? With a camera following me?*

But my expiration date had passed, and I was still alive. Not paralyzed or tethered to a breathing machine. Doing *marathons.* Now, apparently, with a film crew.

It was then I understood the difference between "not dying" and "living."

Not dying was racing until ALS caught up with me. *Living* meant having real dreams—and yes, long-term plans—for the future. Those plans and dreams I had bleached and folded and put away? I had to find the courage to reopen that drawer to think even bigger—because the next part of living was having the audacity to *reach* for what I truly wanted.

It was time. Racing, traveling, and raising money for ALS—the joyful audacity of it all—was necessary. Anything less would be a disservice to myself and to my friends with ALS that I had loved and lost. They would have done anything to have the Hope of life.

Maybe a documentary would bring Hope to those newly diagnosed with ALS. There were plenty of documentaries (and memoirs) tracking the sad, relentless progression of the disease. Definitely important tools for raising awareness of the tragedy of ALS, but did they bring Hope? Triumph of the human spirit, yes. But Hope of survival?

Maybe *this* documentary could be different.

Besides, the timing was too perfect to ignore. Someone recommends a documentary and two weeks later I run into a filmmaker, strike up a conversation and—next thing I know—she's chasing me all over a racecourse with her camera?

My heart pounded thinking of all the possibilities for the marathons, for ALS research, for all of it.

Besides, Jon Blais was clear at the end of his poem: "Whatever you do . . . get it on film."

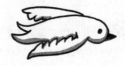

CHAPTER 26

HOW OTHERS LIVE

Kentucky, Connecticut, Colorado, and Hawaii: Marathons #8, #9, #10, and #11 May–October 2019

The Horse Capital Marathon in Kentucky (#8) was one of my more ridiculous ideas. I found the race on a Wednesday. By Friday, we were driving for hours on the curvy mountain roads of West Virginia in the pitch-black night to arrive Saturday morning: the day of the race.

We could have left earlier, but we had an all-day work session with the film-makers. We had decided the documentary would cover the first twenty-one marathons, up through May 2020 at the Prince of Wales Island Marathon in Alaska. The race organizers had invited me to be their guest speaker. A large, remote island in southern Alaska would provide gorgeous scenery for the final race of the film.

That way, we could wrap filming in a year. MJ would do nothing but edit for three months, then apply for film festivals in the fall of 2020 in the "short" category for documentaries under fifty minutes. The short category would avoid competition with feature-length films—which would be far better funded than ours.

The more I got to know MJ and Brian, the more I liked them.

At age twenty-three, Brian had started the Kefa Project to get at-risk Rwandan youth off the streets through soccer. In ten years, Kefa evolved to open a school, support local families, and empower women through micro-businesses. MJ and Brian thoughtfully organized their lives around priorities other than making money: their faith, the kids in Rwanda, and visual storytelling.

I also liked that we could afford them. At least, I hoped so.

The cost of the documentary already stressed me out. Every dollar Team Drea Foundation put toward the film could have been going into a lab for research. We were taking a chance that the film would bring new understanding and fundraising toward ALS, enough to find an eventual cure.

To offset this cost, David and I decided to pay for all marathon travel ourselves. At least potential sponsors and donors wouldn't think we were raising money to fund vacations.

⌘

On race morning in Kentucky, I watched the dark sky soften into pink as the sun cracked the horizon on the Horse Capital Marathon. In the distance, a horse whinnied. The quiet miracle of daily rebirth made me a little weepy. I couldn't believe I would witness a sunrise in every state. *Well, hopefully.*

The race started and finished before I knew it. The wooden fences guided the runners through the rural, rolling hills of horse farms outside Lexington. Although the term "farm" seemed misleading. These were horse *estates*. The wrought-iron gates and sprawling stone manors housed elite horse-racing teams. These were the training grounds of Kentucky Derby champions.

Lifestyles of the Rich and Famous Horses. *Maybe I should ask the horses for money.*

I felt similar pangs of envy at the parking lot for private jets spanning the base of an entire mountain at the Aspen Marathon in Colorado (#10). *How many clinical trials could be funded with this fleet of jets?*

Then I checked myself, because I knew I had the financial freedom to travel to Colorado and race marathons. With a fatal disease. The tenuous beauty of that paradox made me appreciate my privileges all the more.

⌘

Connecticut (#9), before Colorado, had been an odd one. In the pre-race briefing, the race director pointed to a table full of rubber bands. "You pick up a rubber band every time you complete a lap," he said. "On your last lap, ring the bell instead and we will record your time." *Wait, what?*

Welcome to the Mainly Marathons.

Instead of finding 26.2 miles of road to run, the race utilized a slightly-over-one-mile stretch of greenway for participants to go back and forth thirteen times. The rubber bands helped the racers keep track of how many laps each participant completed.

Weaving around small groups of people walking and chatting, I learned that Mainly Marathons racers were a different breed of runner.

Most were significantly older, and the race director said I would be one of the fastest on the course. I didn't really understand until I saw an older man walking slowly with a pronounced stoop. He wore a shirt that read: "This is my _____ marathon." On duct tape over the blank, he had written "992nd." *Wait, what?* Then I spotted a lady walking with a sandwich, then rubber duckies lining the refreshment buffet table (on a racecourse?).

These racers (many aged sixty or older) were going for quantity over speed, fun and connection over competition.

Connecticut was the first race of the Mainly Marathons New England, a seven-day series. Which explained all the walking. And all the RVs in the parking lot.

Their mascot was the Loon, and these racers were, indeed, the Loonies—in the best way possible.

⌘

As soon as I announced my fifty-state goal, my college roommate claimed Hawaii. So, we made the Maui Marathon (#11) our destination for October 2019.

Elizabeth and I were paired as freshman roommates through Davidson College's version of the Myers-Briggs personality test. The room assigners were either gamblers or geniuses because nothing on paper suggested that Elizabeth and I were a match.

My Charleston debutante roommate brought matching powder-blue comforters, complete with dust ruffles and pillow shams, for our twin beds. I had never heard of a debutante, nor had I ever contemplated the existence of a dust ruffle—but I quickly realized its masterful ability to hide the piles of books and notebooks I shoved under the bed.

Elizabeth worked hard and played hard, whereas I just worked. She fixed herself up to go out, while I fixed my backpack up for the library. She still had a higher GPA than me. I may not have been the smartest kid in class, but I could outwork anyone. *The family way.*

Besides, the guilt-ridden good girl in me had to justify the sacrifices my parents made so I could attend an expensive private college. Andy and Sandy were teachers; they didn't own a private jet, like the parents of a girl in my Spanish class. A month before I left for college, we moved back into my childhood home they had kept as a rental property. The sense of financial backsliding hit us all hard. We hadn't worked so hard and sacrificed so much for me to become a drunken idiot on weekends, I told myself. So I stayed in, studied, and missed out on most of the social scene.

Elizabeth accepted my self-righteous non-drinking; I accepted her dust ruffles.

Slowly, we turned into quirky, silly roomies away from home. We sang Backstreet Boys into our hairbrushes, bought a slew of goldfish from Walmart, and named them after our friends. We discovered that Elizabeth's cheerleading skirt was, in fact, shorter than my washcloth.

For the first full year after my diagnosis, Elizabeth wrote a weekly "Throwback Thursday" post on social media recapping the early days of our friendship. (Of course, she had a perfectly curated set of scrapbooks to pull content from.) The birthday box of Lucky Charms where I picked out all the non-marshmallow pieces for her. Our joint twenty-first birthday party with an ice luge, where I finally allowed myself to get drunk.

Since we both assumed I would die soon, her living tribute felt extra special. I had seen so many people post photos and memories to social media after a friend passed away. We don't celebrate our friendships enough while we are alive. *We might not have taken this trip together if I wasn't dying*, I thought as our plane touched down in Maui.

MJ and Brian were filming the West Coast figure-skating circuit but had a perfectly timed week off to pop over to Hawaii.

"What do you want Elizabeth and me to—um—like, talk about? What do you want us to say on camera?" I asked MJ. They planned to tag along on the famous Road to Hana to see the waterfalls.

"Just be yourselves," MJ said. "Forget we're here."

Easier said than done with a camera sticking out from the back seat. Most of our filming so far had been sit-down interviews. Or marathons, where I only had to huff and puff on the trike.

In the age of reality TV, full of shouting matches ending in wine thrown in someone's face, I worried that two reasonably sane, sober, occasionally silly college roommates would bore the audience. In this version of reality, my slow speech failed to even deliver a decent sound bite.

My fears were confirmed when MJ put down the camera after asking a few questions and listening to us reminisce. Our stories sounded awkwardly formal. I obviously had no idea what I had gotten myself into with a documentary. I was just a normal thirtysomething accidentally cast into the leading role of an unfolding drama involving ALS, a trike, and some self-inflicted marathons. I was a bad actor. I didn't know my lines. Heck, I didn't even know the ending.

❧

"Can we go out to the beach?" I asked MJ that night. "There's something I want to talk about."

She looked at me quizzically. "Sure."

I was afraid to say anything else. Afraid I would cry, and therefore be unintelligible.

We found a semi-quiet stretch of sand. I plopped down on a towel. We looked out at the water and the island of Lanai. The setting sun had slipped behind clouds, but the water still shimmered.

"What do you want to talk about?" MJ asked, aiming the camera at me.

"Death," I said, grinning that smile of mine that holds tears back. I couldn't say anything else for a while. *How am I going to get through this?* I swallowed hard.

MJ waited. The documentary was not about fame. The documentary was an opportunity to talk to the world about how shitty ALS is—but also, how beautiful life is. How precious, how fragile.

"When was the last time you were able to get in the water?" she asked.

I recounted my snorkeling attempt in Turks and Caicos, where the undertow knocked me down in knee-deep water and revealed how weak I had become. How David and I spent the rest of the trip sitting on the sand, looking out at the water. *Kind of like this. But never, ever could I have imagined this journey back then.*

I told her how, at the time, I didn't know what to do with my remains after I was gone—whether to be buried or cremated.

I paused, trying to get my voice under control.

"Life is so temporary," I said slowly. "But it always continues. Maybe if I had my ashes scattered, then maybe I would become a shell. Or a fish. Or a shark." I smiled, remembering my decision on the beach in Turks and Caicos. *A speck of me, anyway.*

"Do you feel like you have peace about death?" she asked.

I nodded slowly, choking back the sobs that threatened my voice. I wanted desperately to be able to say the next thing.

"What really matters is what we choose to do with the time we have," I said. How we live. No matter how long that might be.

That was what I had learned from Jon Blais, from the horse estates, the jets in Aspen, from the Loonies completing hundreds of marathons together.

That was what I needed to say.

⁂

The next morning, we set off on a catamaran for snorkeling. I told Brian about the snorkeling scare in Turks and Caicos—and that I would not be getting in the water.

"No worries. It'll be beautiful. We'll grab some B-roll footage of Maui. It's fine."

Oh, but how I desperately wanted to try snorkeling again. It had been such a blow to give up swimming in the ocean. Plus, I had been swimming twice a week, for what, three years now? I felt stronger than I had since before the diagnosis.

I want to try.

We headed out to Molokini, a partially submerged volcanic crater in the shape of a half moon. Our guides promised that the cove would protect us from the strong winds and currents crossing the channel. I wasn't paying much attention as a guide strapped a yellow, loose-fitting float belt around my waist. My eyes were fixed on Molokini, which rose up like the spine of some giant underwater sea creature. Waves slammed into the smooth crater wall.

I still want to try.

Hesitantly, I leaned forward to put my face mask and snorkel into the water and kicked off. The float belt immediately lifted my butt and stomach to the surface of the water. My head was angled down. I resembled a skewered shrimp.

I immediately tasted saltwater in my snorkel and panicked. *Shit, shit, shit! I can't aspirate salt water!* I pictured the saltwater spraying into my lungs—who knew what kind of pneumonia *that* would cause? Kicking furiously, I tried to force my legs down and lift my head. My head cleared the surface but there was still water in the snorkel. Treading water, I tried to empty the snorkel one-handed. I looked around. Everyone had their heads down, snorkels up—looking at whatever was below.

Don't freak out. You're a strong swimmer. You're just getting used to the snorkel. More than anything, I wanted to prove to myself I could do it. To prove that ALS wasn't winning, and certainly not in Hawaii.

I tried again. The same thing: butt up, head down, water in snorkel. Definite rising panic.

This would be a pretty dumb way to die.

Elizabeth was nearby, so I tried waving to her under the water. She waved back and smiled through her snorkel, looking back at the fish. Finally, MJ realized I was in trouble.

"Brian!" she yelled. "Help!" Closest to the boat, Brian grabbed a boogie board. I grabbed on, feeling ridiculous.

"Sorry, I didn't realize you were in distress," Elizabeth said, as she towed the board and me back to the boat. "I wasn't sure if you were reaching for me or pushing me away."

Back safely on board, I insisted the others go back out. "I'm fine, I'm fine."

Closing my eyes behind sunglasses and facing the water, frustrated tears ran down my cheeks. I knew I shouldn't feel embarrassed, but I was. I hated all the fuss, the accommodations made for me. After all that swimming, I still couldn't snorkel.

As everyone piled back into the boat, I shut down my internal pity party. *You're still in Hawaii, dammit.*

"Are you going to go back out?" MJ asked on camera as the boat headed back toward shore for our next stop at the reef known as Turtle Town.

"Nah," I said. "I'll stay." Safer for my body. Safer for my ego.

The guides assured me the water would be calmer in Turtle Town. No float belt, just the boogie board. "And I'll be on alert," Elizabeth said.

Okay, fine. I'll try again.

Back in the water, I made tentative strokes. I leaned in. *See? I* can *swim after all.*

Above the reef of Turtle Town, I threw my arm over the boogie board and Elizabeth clamped her hand over my arm. All we had to do was put our faces in the water. Two college roomies, just hanging out. Not a cloud in the sky, not a dust ruffle in sight.

A dozen turtles floated around the base of the reef, completely unconcerned with the humans above. Rays of light filtered down onto their massive shells. Graceful, gentle giants, rising and falling on the waves and the current. My body relaxed and awe took over.

My mind connected back to my conversation with MJ on the beach. *I could become a turtle. A speck of me, anyway. Think of the adventures I could go on.*

Besides, I already knew how to swim.

CHAPTER 27

CRUNCH TIME

From the moment I launched my fifty-state challenge, there was one obvious choice for my final race: the Boston Marathon.

Boston is the longest-running, most prestigious marathon in the world. A runner is not permitted to merely "sign up" for Boston; rather, they must qualify (aka "Boston Qualify" or "BQ") based on a finish time from another marathon.

The Boston Athletic Association (BAA) dictates qualifying times based on age group and gender categories of male and female, as well as the newly introduced nonbinary category in 2022.[1] Even with a challenging standard, too many runners meet the threshold, so each year the *actual* qualifying time is faster than posted.

If a runner can't qualify by time, they can participate by fundraising for one of two dozen approved charities.[2] Roughly one-fifth of the marathon's spots (approximately 6,000 entries)[3] are reserved each year for charities, sponsors, vendors, licensees, consultants, municipal officials, local running clubs, and marketers. These entries are considered "invitational" by the BAA.[4]

I knew I'd have to apply to race Boston, because my trike wasn't a standard adaptive "vehicle," like a push-rim wheelchair or a handcycle. But when I declared my fifty-marathon goal, it felt too early to approach the BAA about participating. After all, I had more than forty left. *Who knows, they may change the rules by the time I get there. Or, more likely, I'll die before I get to fifty.*

But I began to pay more attention to my race times in order to strengthen my argument to the BAA—and I had already achieved a 3:35 BQ-time in four marathons. I just needed to keep racing and keep the pace up to add more BQ times to my argument for Boston to include me.

Pennsylvania: Marathon #12
November 2019

The Philadelphia Marathon had been my first half marathon, eight years before.

In November, I returned to Philly for marathon #12. Even though I loved my trike and felt my pride growing with each marathon, I crumbled with jealousy remembering myself as that newly minted runner back in 2011. She was so innocent, so full of wonder at what her body could do and what could be possible if she just worked at it. *Work harder.*

My mood was on the skids anyway. After hosting our last fundraiser of the year, I was spent. I had nothing left to tackle the mountain of thank-you notes, tax receipts, and end-of-year bookkeeping. I definitely had nothing left for Christmas cards and general merrymaking.

Instead of Productive Andrea, Exhausted Andrea spent three days angrily watching the Kavanaugh Supreme Court hearings and playing Sudoku. My procrastination response shows up with a vengeance when I'm tired and over-whelmed. I recognized the pattern but could not shake it.

I had officially shut down.

I arrived at the Philadelphia start line mad at myself, mad at the frigid, windy weather, and super mad about my assigned bike escort. Bike escorts are usually kind and well-meaning, but I *always* resented having a babysitter.

My preferred bike escorts are quiet and stay behind me, available only if I need something. But this guy was hell-bent on *really* escorting me. Every few seconds, he yelled "on your left!" completely startling runners from behind. Shaken out of their running daze, the runners tripped trying to get out of our way, apologizing the whole time. *How embarrassing.*

Helpful though, I admitted a few miles in. At least I wasn't getting stuck behind packs of runners with music blasting through their headphones, oblivious to the pint-sized trike behind them. I was faster with the bike escort in front of me. I pedaled harder to keep up. Like, I didn't want to inconvenience *him* by slowing *him* down. By the time I spotted David and his family in the crowd, I was smiling again.

I wouldn't hit a PR, but I *might* hit my BQ time of 3:35.

The cold rain had soaked through two layers of leggings, my gloves, my shoes, and both pairs of socks. *The faster you finish, the faster you're out of these miserable clothes.*

I aimed the trike toward the Art Museum, those famous "Rocky Balboa" stairs, and pedaled as hard as I could. Two miles to go.

I clocked in at 3:36:27. Frustratingly close. But at least my smile was back . . . for the moment.

❧

After Philadelphia, I returned to the black hole of sadness. Not just crabbiness from the holiday pressure, but a stare-at-the-wall kind of misery.

I had always set ambitious goals for myself. The bigger the better so that the fear of failure would drive me to achieve whatever I set out to do—whether college finals or a half-distance triathlon. I pushed and pushed myself toward achievement.

Until ALS.

When I believed I had a short time to live, my true priorities became clear: David, family, ALS research. But as time passed and I stayed alive, I found myself bogged down in the grind of life. Like a regular person again, but with frustrating limitations. My default formula wasn't working anymore. Even with thirty-seven remaining marathons still hanging over my head.

No one gave me a medal for doing the foundation's bookkeeping. No one cared when I launched the next fundraiser. No boss, no accountability. Without the external factors I used previously to light a fire under my butt, I felt nothing to push against, nothing to strive toward. Team Drea was a volunteer gig, so I had no one to stop me from playing sixteen games of Sudoku or binge-watching the latest Keeping Up with the Whoever Housewives of Wherever. *You don't have a job. No one is expecting anything from you.*

So, when this voice chimed in, I did "nothing," which cued the next phase of my demented process. Self-torment. *You ungrateful sloth. You have been given the gift of time, and this is what you choose to do with it? What do you think your dead friends would have to say about that?*

That usually led to crying, then more Sudoku and Housewives for the rest of the evening to block out the sounds of damning recrimination in my head.

Oh, and let's not forget, part three: the glowing promise to start fresh in the morning.

Fresh Morning Me would feel so guilty about yesterday's Sloth Me that I would throw the covers off the bed and attack the day. While the scheme worked in the beginning, a deeper level of self-sabotage began to whisper soothingly: *The new Housewives is on. Don't you deserve a little downtime? You do have ALS, you know.*

Then there I was again, watching TV and squandering away the precious life I was never supposed to live to see anyway.

A few years prior, when I had exhibited this pattern, I enlisted the help of a life coach. *Like a therapist for my to-do list,* I thought. But her insights turned out to be much more profound.

After listening to me complain this time, Beth pulled out a fresh sheet of paper and drew a perfect sine wave. *Up, down, up, down.*

"I think you want to live your entire life up here," she said, pointing to the top of the curve.

I cracked up. *Duh. Yes, that is exactly what I want. What's the problem?* But with her drawing, I realized how unrealistic that was—for anyone—ALS or not.

"Your value as a person is not defined by what you do in life, you know," Beth said.

I cocked an eyebrow. "Say what?"

She said it again, slower and adding emphasis. "Your *value* is not defined by your *productivity*. Your value is who you *are* as a *person*."

I paused.

"I get it," I said. (I did not get it.)

All the way home, I turned it over in my head. My family's pride was productivity. We pushed, and we were proud for doing so. *Work harder.* The end.

So, what was all this "value is not defined by your productivity" business? We all have value, because we are all unique and special in our own way? It is who we are, not what or how much we do?

I shrugged. *Sure, okay. If you say so.*

But I did not get it.

⊰⊱

Over the years I'd worked with Beth, I had made some progress in cutting myself some slack.

"Andrea, Team Drea is so much more than just the money we raise," our board member Doug said. "You inspire people to be brave. That is also our mission, even if we can't quantify it."

Everyone else on the board agreed.

So I started there with a small change, a small release of pressure. I stopped sweating our year-end financial goals for the foundation. And in the letting go, I noticed the goals were met that year. And again the next. No freak-outs required.

I will say that Beth gave me a *look* when I told her about the fifty marathons and the documentary.

"I know, I know," I said. "But I'm learning to trust myself. This feels different."

We talked through strategies to take some work off my plate to make room for more races, which included an intern—who wiped out a six-month backlog of projects in less than a month. She took over the internal bookkeeping for me, updated our website, and posted regularly on social media. Although I could no longer brag to donors that "Team Drea has no paid staff so all your money goes straight to ALS research," I felt so much lighter and knew that we would do more good with more help.

Since I had been doing so well, the backslide into this Beth-identified rut pattern "up, down, up, down" after Philadelphia had caught me off guard. How ridiculous to complain about traveling to Hawaii, the ability to do multiple marathons, having two successful fundraisers, and filming a documentary. *Cue the guilt.*

But I was exhausted. Exhaustion usually leads me to a loss of perspective.

Between strangled sobs, I admitted to Beth how much time I wasted with reality TV and Sudoku. In all the time we had worked together, I had never cried like this.

"It's worse than ever. I'm, like, *refusing* to thrive," I said, sniffling.

"Remember," she said, "your value is not defined by how productive you are."

I stopped wiping my nose. *Here we go. This BS again.*

"Honestly, I've never understood that. I've always had pride in working hard."

"But when we focus on *being* instead of *doing*, we don't need to define our value by how productive we are. *Who we are* shapes what we choose to do."

I mulled that over.

"*Being* requires doing, yes. But in ways that don't translate easily to a to-do list," Beth said. "Like the way you inspire people, going out of your way for a friend, listening to your husband's bad day at work, being present to appreciate the life you have and world you exist in. That is the *being* translating to *doing*. And yes, self-care is part of that."

In other words, I could never *do* enough to convince myself that I *was* enough.

At the end of our session, Beth walked me to my car. She put my walker in the back seat and leaned over to hug me.

"You are a cheerleader of humanity," she said.

I finally got it.

Alabama: Marathon #13
December 2019

With Beth's words ringing in my ears, David and I flew to Alabama for my final race of the year: the Rocket City Marathon (#13).

Who knew NASA built rockets in Huntsville, Alabama? I surely didn't.

Be present was my race mantra. Instead of looking for pacers in order to gauge my time, I resumed my city tours. The course circled the grounds of the US Space and Rocket Center, passing the first satellites and moon rovers displayed outside. Never would I have explored this town without this race, this goal, this disease.

Pedaling along, lost in thought, I spotted the 3:30 pacer. *Wait, what?* I assumed they were long gone.

I made a deal with myself. As long as I remained present in the moment, I could go as fast as I wanted. *Stay present.*

My focus sharpened. I connected with my muscles, proud of them. *Thank you for still being here.* Remembering my Pilates techniques, I tuned into each muscle in the chain, feeling each engage in succession. I could feel the gratitude in my body.

Suddenly, the off-road patch the race organizers had warned me about came into view. They had sent me photos of this stretch of course, about a half mile in length, a shortcut through the trees to get to the adjacent arboretum.

"It'll be fine," I had said, and then forgot all about it.

Slowing to a crawl as I navigated around tree roots and across slippery pine needles, I looked up to see the 3:30 pacer pass by, sign still bouncing along. *That's okay,* I told myself. *Stay present.*

Back on pavement, I willed myself not to take off. *Hold steady until 5K left, then you can sprint. Your feelings about this race will not be dictated by your time.*

At the mile 23 marker, I picked up the pace. Just for fun, just to see what I could do. Grinning, I passed the 3:30 pacer for the final time.

The Rocket City Marathon finished *inside* the downtown convention center, by way of a loading dock. I was so far ahead of my usual finish time that David hadn't even arrived yet. No matter. I collected my astronaut-themed medal and cruised around the convention center floor searching for the source of the delicious smell that permeated the building. *Popcorn!* Hot, buttery, salty popcorn. David found me in a corner, munching away happily.

"Whoa!" he exclaimed. "Where did you come from?" He leaned down to kiss me.

When we checked my official time, I had a new PR: 3:29:05, besting my Horse Capital Marathon time by fifty-four seconds.

Add it to my future argument for Boston—I now had five BQ-qualifying times. *Not that it matters*, I reminded myself.

Afterward, I bought myself the perfect Christmas present: a wooden US map with the states outlined, complete with hooks for each state medal. After finishing each marathon, I colored in the state with neon chalk marker and hung its medal below. I stared at that map often, imagining the future races and what the terrain and cities would be like. For the ones I'd completed, the hanging medals triggered memories that I alone carried.

No one could take these memories from me, not even ALS.

By the beginning of 2020, I'd completed most of the southern states within driving distance. A satisfying cluster of bright orange, pink, and green states appeared on my map.

But the map was entirely blank west of the Mississippi River, except for Texas, Colorado, and Hawaii. *Time to remedy that.*

Arizona: Marathon #14
January 2020

This one feels like cheating. I laughed to myself, whizzing past yet another cactus.

The Buckeye Marathon (#14) consisted of twenty miles on a very straight highway, pitched slightly downhill. I practically could have rolled down the entire course without pedaling.

No question that wheels and gravity helped me speed downhill, which might seem unfair to other runners.

But I wished my trike had a sign on the back: "Don't worry, you'll catch me on the uphill!"

Because, as easy as the downhills were, each uphill came at a cost.

Gravity worked hard against me going uphill. I also had an additional thirty pounds of trike that waited for me to let up my effort so it could roll backward. As I slogged each climb in my lowest gear, the runner I had just passed on the downhill would catch me—even if they were walking.

When I finished the Buckeye Marathon with a new PR of 3:17:22, I was slightly disappointed. I enjoyed sneaking up on my PR race by race and beating it by a few seconds or a minute. This gave me something to strive for. The Arizona time would be hard to beat again.

Go figure—only I would be disappointed by success.

CHAPTER 28

ANDREA THE FILMMAKER

Louisiana: Marathon #15
February 2020

As an urban explorer with a documentary film crew in tow, I could not wait for the marathon in New Orleans—a city I'd always wanted to visit. In my eagerness, I packed way too much into our schedule. And subsequently turned the long weekend into a nightmare.

After our early-morning flight on Friday, MJ and Brian picked me up from our hotel. I had received an Adventure grant from Team Gleason to travel to New Orleans, so Team Gleason HQ would be the first stop on our schedule.

Steve Gleason is an NFL hero to both the city of New Orleans and to the ALS community. Gleason is famous for one play with the New Orleans Saints—a blocked punt so memorable it is enshrined as a bronze statue outside the Superdome. In one of the opening plays of the Saints's first home game nearly two years after Katrina devastated the city, Gleason blocked a punt that his teammate recovered in the end zone for a touchdown. The Saints won the game and went all the way to the NFC Championship that season, restoring hope to the battered city. The statue is titled *Rebirth*.

In 2011, Steve Gleason was diagnosed with ALS at the age of thirty-four. The Team Gleason Foundation has provided communication and medical equipment worth more than $20 million to people with ALS, helping to improve their quality of life and maintain their independence. The Steve Gleason Act, signed into law in 2015 with unanimous votes from both houses of Congress, ensures that expensive communication devices, like eye-gaze technology, are covered by Medicare. A couple of weeks before our trip to New Orleans, Steve received the Congressional Gold Medal for his contributions to ALS awareness.

When the 2016 *Gleason* documentary made it into theaters, Julie and I drove to Boston to watch it with ALS TDI staff. While the audience sniffled or shed a tear during particularly raw scenes, such as Steve reading letters to his unborn son, those of us with firsthand ALS experience spent the entire movie bawling.

While I appreciated the film's uplifting message about the triumph of the human spirit, the film hit too close to home. I couldn't unsee the scenes of Steve's body shriveling away, or the exhausted look on his wife Michel's face as her role of "spouse" transformed into "caregiver."

David and my mom had planned to see it together the next day, but I forbade them to go. It would have been too much.

But now, four years later, I knew my path wasn't following the typical ALS trajectory. Our documentary would be different, but I thought Steve Gleason's work and tagline of "No White Flags" fit in perfectly with the message I wanted to share with the audience. *Besides, if I could just grab onto his coattails, it would give our film more legitimacy . . .*

We toured the Team Gleason House, a nursing home wing equipped with technology for people living with ALS. Elevators, window blinds, doors, and televisions could be controlled with eye-gaze technology. I thought a documentary scene there would be powerful. It could call attention to everyday conveniences lost to ALS, while instilling hope for a world where that technology could be built in to preserve independence.

But we didn't have the right permissions. Obviously, the nursing staff wouldn't allow us to film their residents for privacy reasons. I hadn't reached out in advance. *I should have known better. Ugh!*

Then the race officials issued a final no for press passes for MJ and Brian to have unrestricted access to the start and finish line areas.

"But what about filming in general?" MJ asked. "Do we have permission for that?"

"I can't stop you from filming from a public sidewalk, can I?" the liaison snapped. *Is that a yes?*

By lunchtime, I felt a lump of frustration in my throat as we navigated the clogged streets of the French Quarter near Bourbon Street.

A text came from my friend Liz in a bar across town: "Where are you?"

Shit! Liz was going to introduce me—and hopefully the filmmakers—to Steve Gleason. Even though Liz had already told me she could *not* use her personal friendship with Steve to ask about filming, my brain said, *If she could just meet MJ and Brian, see how cool they are, and maybe she'd invite them to meet Steve—what an amazing addition to our film!*

On the way to the bar to meet Liz, MJ and Brian discussed yet another glitch in our filming schedule. Traffic kept crawling. It was all too much. All too important, all happening at once. I couldn't *do* anything to fix it. I kneaded my hands together, willing myself not to cry.

When we parked more than a half-hour late, I couldn't take off my seat belt, my hands were shaking so badly. *Forget ALS. I'm paralyzed by my own stupidity, my lack of planning—or was it overplanning?*

"Uh, can you guys give us a second?" David said to the filmmakers. MJ and Brian lowered their cameras and nodded. They went into the bar.

Shaking, wailing, and so embarrassed, I heaved sobs into my hands. *Too much. Too much.*

"Just breathe, babe. You're okay. Just breathe," David said soothingly, stroking my knee. He looked bewildered. He had absolutely no idea what had happened.

Eventually, I pulled myself together. I had to. With my face a blotchy mess, we walked into the bar. The filmmakers and Liz were seated at the first table by the window. They had a front-row seat to my meltdown.

"ALS is a bitch, ain't it?" Liz said, enveloping me in a hug. I couldn't answer. *Not ALS. Just me being a dumbass, trying to coordinate my life to fit a documentary.*

In the end, David and I did meet Steve Gleason and his wife, Michel, at their house. The filmmakers weren't invited. I didn't get the dramatic movie moment I wanted, but I *did* get to thank Steve for giving hope to those of us with ALS. My voice cracked with emotion, and true sincerity.

Quiet on the car ride back to our hotel, I looked up at the moon. *I am getting out of the filmmaking business*, I thought. No more tours, no more trying to make scenes happen. *We might end up with a boring documentary, but at least it will be real.*

And I might have half a chance of remaining sane.

⊲⊚⊳

The next morning, we discovered the new bike pump had the wrong fitting for the trike. About an hour before the race. When I heard the sickening sound of air escaping the tire, the lump in my throat from the day before returned.

The tire was half deflated before I yelled, "Stop!"

David looked up at me with murder in his eyes. "You *told* me to do this!" he snarled.

All caught on video, of course.

Maybe I can do it on two wheels, I thought as I triked through the halls and into the elevator toward the hotel lobby. My back wheel was deflated. *Maybe if I just lean forward a little?* Ridiculous. But we were late to the start. We just had to figure it out on the way.

"Excuse us, excuse us." David's usually friendly tone was a growl as we cut through the crowd.

Then I spotted our savior.

"David!" I yelled.

"What?"

"Bike!" I pointed.

A bike marshal for the race stood over by the sidewalk. David started sprinting. I followed.

"Oh, thank you, thank you!" I said as the man knelt, filling my back tire with an emergency CO_2 cartridge. As soon as I heard the lifesaving air inflating the tire, the first real smile of the day lit up my face. *Hope.*

⊲⊚⊳

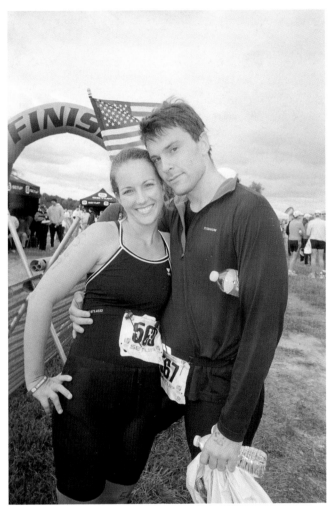

Andrea and David Peet. First-ever sprint triathlon in 2011. Andrea is ready for another; David thought one was enough. *Photo courtesy of Dr. Dave Peet.*

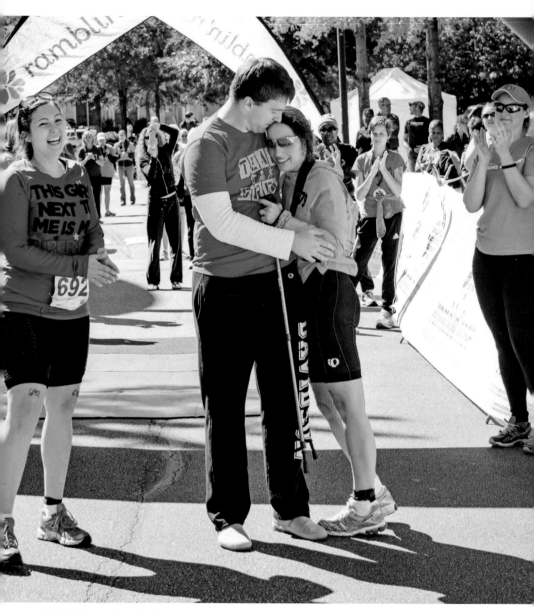

Julie Wesner, Andrea's childhood friend, David Peet, and Andrea Lytle Peet at the finish line of the 2014 Ramblin' Rose Triathlon. The spark that changed everything. *Photo courtesy of Tamara Lackey.*

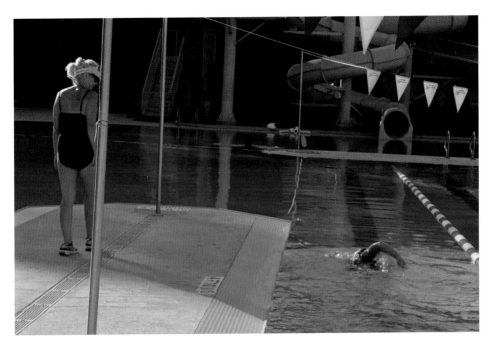

ABOVE: Andrea and her ever-vigilant, ever-supportive mom, Sandy Lytle, during a swim workout. *Photo courtesy of Brian Beckman and Miriam McSpadden, from* Go On, Be Brave. RIGHT: Dr. Rick Bedlack, Andrea's neurologist at Duke, and Andrea in 2019. Dr. Bedlack reserves his best outfits for ALS Clinic days. *Photo courtesy of Sandy Lytle.*

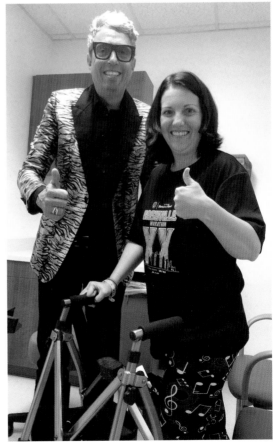

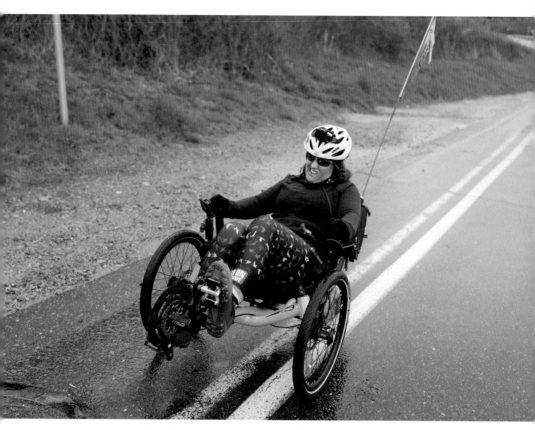

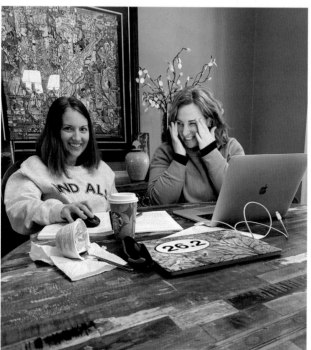

ABOVE: Andrea fighting the freezing rain on Purgatory Road in Newport, Rhode Island (#27). *Photo courtesy of Brian Beckman and Miriam McSpadden, from* Go On, Be Brave. LEFT: Andrea with co-author Meredith Atwood during an in-person edit session in December 2022. A marathon of a different kind. *Photo courtesy of Stella Atwood.*

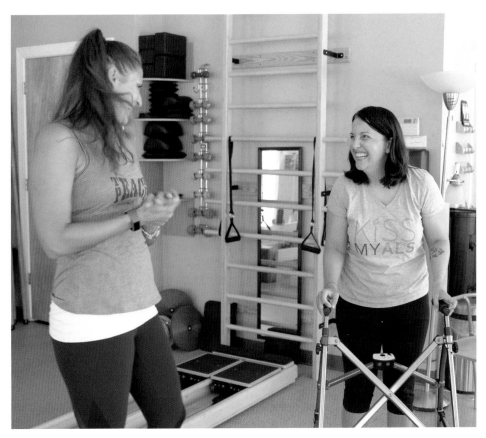

Andrea with her Pilates-based physical therapist, Mischa Decker. *Photo courtesy of Brian Beckman and Miriam McSpadden, from* Go On, Be Brave.

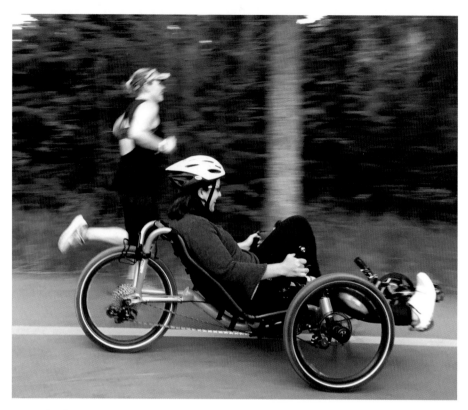

ABOVE: Andrea racing with friend Katie Brooks Elliott in Aspen, Colorado (#10). *Photo courtesy of John Peet and Molly Rosenblatt.* BELOW: Andrea receives a Boston Marathon medal from Ryan Auster, her college rowing teammate. *Photo courtesy of Brian Beckman and Miriam McSpadden, from* Go On, Be Brave.

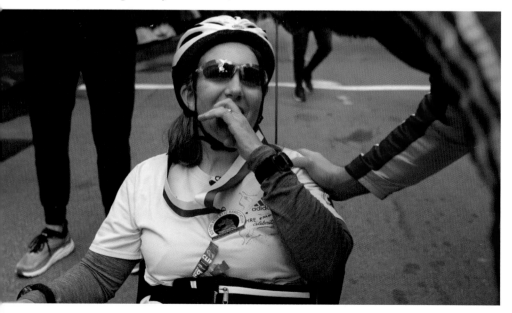

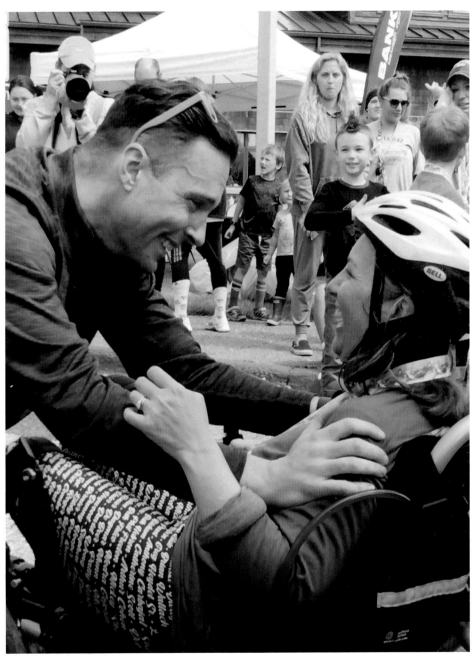

Andrea and David Peet at the finish line in Alaska (#50). *Photo courtesy of Mark McCready.*

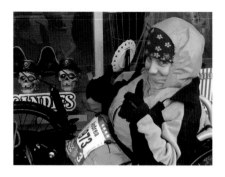

ABOVE: Andrea braving the elements at the Yuengling Shamrock Marathon in Virginia Beach, Virginia (#2). *Photo courtesy of David Peet.* BELOW: Andrea with an arm full of swallow tattoos, one for every year living with ALS. *Photo courtesy of Brian Beckman and Miriam McSpadden.*

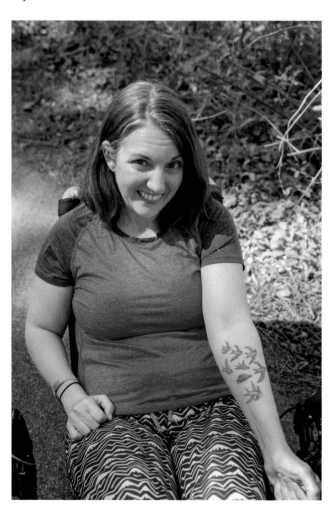

Three hours later, I felt like the worst kind of hypocrite.

The grateful adrenaline had long since worn off. *I tell people to just be grateful for what their bodies can do. Hello, my name is Andrea, and I am fucking miserable.*

My left leg was not working.

No matter how hard I concentrated on straight alignment, my left leg crossed the centerline of the trike like a drunk driver. It fell in and over with each pedal stroke. I noticed the issue every race, but this time the filmmakers had mounted a GoPro to the center post coming up between my feet. My left calf banged into the camera with every stroke. Of course, it hadn't happened when we tested the setup before the race—my legs were strong and fresh then. But seventeen miles into the marathon, the camera was scraping a hole into my floppy left leg. Like, literally—a *hole*.

Then came the bridges.

Below-sea-level New Orleans is pancake flat, but there were several bridges over canals or highways. On the elevation profile for the race, they looked like small ant hills—six of them lined up. Three up, three back. Yesterday, on our drive of the course, the little hills had seemed innocuous.

Dammit, I thought now, cursing Yesterday-in-the-Car Andrea.

My left leg flopped over, every strike of the exposed flesh shooting barbs of pain up my leg. Throw in an unnaturally steep hill. *Dammit all.*

At mile 18, I saw the 3:35 pacer coming toward me. *Dammit.* He had already reached the turnaround point, just a bit ahead.

As I said before, exhaustion usually caused a loss of perspective. I became determined to catch the pacer for another BQ time.

Slogging my way through the crowd, I could tell I was making progress. I could see his bouncing sign. *Yes! It's working!* I kept pushing, reeling him in. *Make this count,* I told myself. *Fight harder!*

The instant I passed the pacer, I felt a burst of elation, followed by searing pain from my leg bashing against the GoPro. A yelp of pain escaped my throat. *Focus, dammit.*

I maintained my lead over the pacer until we hit the next bridge.

As I started up the hill, the trike slowed to a dead stop and threatened to roll backward. The pacer cruised past, oblivious that I was racing him. Demoralized, I knew it was over.

I had no power remaining in my legs. My left calf screamed in pain. My vision of a BQ time evaporated. From the hills of Austin, I knew how to get over this bridge—half stroke, clamp on brakes, reset, half stroke—repeat. I could do it. I *would* do it, but the BQ time was gone.

Why does it even matter? It doesn't, Andrea. 3:35 is a stupid standard you made up. Who knew the actual time standard the BAA would use, or if they would even allow the trike?

Cresting the top of the bridge, I took a deep breath and let the trike coast with the pressure off. *When will I learn?*

This journey was not about BQ-ing marathons.

The journey was not about *doing* marathons. Beth's words came back: "The doing doesn't shape who you are. Who you *are* shapes what you choose to *do*."

Against all odds, I am alive. It's not really that complicated.

I cracked up laughing right there in the trike.

⁂

At my next Pilates session with Mischa, I enlisted her expertise in the mis-alignment of my left knee.

"See?" I said. "No matter what I do, it's like my whole knee goes inward." I pedaled the trike on the indoor trainer I had brought to my appointment.

"Yeah, but it's really your whole thigh. It's coming from all the way up here," Mischa said, tapping on my glutes. "So when you go to full extension, you get that inward rotation."

She had exercises for that, of course.

We began dedicating sessions to strengthening my glutes and external rotation of my hips and outer thighs. In the pool, I worked on my "frog" moves, opening up my hips. My seventy-five-year-old mother had the flexibility of a gymnast compared to me. I hadn't realized how tight and stiff I had become.

At least I had thirty-five more marathons to work on it.

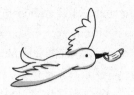

CHAPTER 29

HOPE GETS COVID

Mississippi and Arkansas: Marathons #16 and #17
February–Early March 2020

KAA-CHUNK!

I hit a pothole, and the trike chain and my legs froze mid-stride. Ten miles into the Mississippi Blues Marathon (#16) on Leap Day, February 29, 2020, I was officially stuck.

Worse yet, I still had Arkansas (#17) the next day.

So much for my brilliant plan to save money by doubling up on marathons. *Do not panic*, I instructed myself. *This is not another New Orleans.*

I coasted into a shady patch of grass and craned my neck, trying to see the chain under the frame. No go. The only thing left to do was dig my phone out of my sweaty leggings.

"What? Stuck?" David said as I tried to explain on speakerphone.

With all the road closures, he said he would have to run—as in yes, run—over to meet me. He was in downtown Jackson, four miles away. He was a good runner, but it would still take some time.

We hung up and I closed my eyes. I arched my back to stretch out the tightness from sitting in one position. When I opened them again, a parade of puffy white clouds marched across the bright blue sky.

A reminder that time was passing. Time to get serious.

One busted marathon, *fine*. But two busted marathons? No, that I could not handle. We needed to get the trike fixed fast, get out of Mississippi, and drive the four hours to Little Rock before packet pickup closed at 6 P.M. *It's okay. We can come back to Mississippi.*

While I waited on David, I searched on my phone for a nearby bike shop. Got it. Oh wait, a *trike* shop! A half hour away—the only one in all of Mississippi. Lucky.

David arrived, sweating and out of breath from sprinting four miles. I stared at him, never more in love than at that moment.

"You okay?" He seemed surprised I wasn't crying.

"Yeah. It's okay. We can come back to Mississippi," I said, echoing the phrase my brain had been repeating.

"Hell, no. We're getting you back on the road." *Wait, what?*

He lay down in the grass to get a better view of the chain. Fifteen minutes later, he was covered in grease and had used all the curse words he knew, plus a few invented ones. The chain was back on, but the trike wouldn't shift. The pothole had bent the derailleur.

"Can you do the race without shifting—like at all?" he asked, wiping sweat from his forehead and leaving a greasy smudge. *How can I say no to that cute smudge?*

All I could do was try. What did I have to lose? Hope? "I will do it," I said, and I took off, adding with a wave, "I love you!"

I plowed through the rest of the race like the trike was on fire. Or maybe that was my quads. But I was proud of my slowest time ever: 4:59:39.

⟡

"It's *okay*, I promise," I said to David, as he put the trike in the car.

There was no way we'd make it to Arkansas in time for the packet pickup.*

---

* Packet pickup is required for most races, usually with no exceptions. You have to arrive by the time it closes, or you don't race. This is how they account for who is racing the next day. While some races allow pickup the day of, most big races usually do the day or days prior.

"Don't worry about it. I've already done one marathon this weekend."

But that's not David's way. Let's be honest—it wasn't mine either. So at 2 P.M., with the trike fixed, David sped toward Little Rock. We had exactly four hours to make it to packet pickup.

When the blue lights flashed behind us, we lost more time and gained a speeding ticket. *We still have time. We got this . . . maybe.*

Nothing was around us for miles, just one straight highway bisecting the cotton and soybean fields, stretched out in all directions as far as our eyes could see. I wanted to see America, and this was it. I settled back in the seat, still in my sweaty Mississippi race clothes.

On the radio, we listened to a report about a new virus spreading fast around the globe.

Days earlier, the US Centers for Disease Control had held a briefing and warned that the public should brace for the eventual spread of COVID-19 across the country.

Surely not, I thought, and closed my eyes for a nap. I slept until David swung wildly into a parking spot at packet pickup with ten minutes to spare.

The next day, I secured #17 at the Little Rock Marathon.

~~California: Marathon #18~~
March 2020

The SoCal Marathon was set for March 21, 2020.

On March 11, the World Health Organization declared COVID-19 a global pandemic.

Ten days away from SoCal, I refused to cancel. "My breathing is *normal*," I snapped when David suggested that I—in particular—should, you know, maybe consider not getting on a plane to California right now.

The governor of California spared us further argument by prohibiting gatherings of more than 250 people. The race was canceled.

I glued myself to news coverage of our country spiraling into crisis. I watched coverage of people suddenly losing their livelihoods. People experiencing abject terror about a deadly disease that could strike anyone at any time. Commentary about how scary it felt to not know what was coming next. All of it, all the news, felt . . . familiar.

Yes, on a totally different scale—a global economy and millions of lives were at stake—but I felt a scary camaraderie. *I know this fear.* And that, oddly, comforted me.

I looked for signs that had saved my sanity before—in the dark times after I was diagnosed. I retraced my steps, looking for the calm I had felt. I recalled the sun on my face as I walked out of the hospital. Walking, talking, eating with my husband and my parents. *I am okay, right this moment. Be grateful. Love your people.*

We were privileged and fortunate. David could work from home. His job wasn't in danger. My parents were mostly retired. We didn't have to instantaneously figure out childcare or remote schooling.

When our gym closed, my parents bought a recumbent trike. I was *thrilled.* Each time Mom had complained about her puny quads, I'd said, "Well, that's why you need a trike." Each time Dad had complained about his balance getting worse, I'd said, "Well, that's why you need a trike."

Overjoyed, I met them at the bike shop to pick out their trike: a silver Catrike Expedition with a chain tensioner to accommodate their height differences, making it easier to switch between riders. Two matching helmets. Two pairs of bike shoes.

All perfect—until we got to the parking lot. Then I overheard Dad talking to the bike mechanic.

"Yeah, I think this will be good. That way we can ride with Andrea so she won't need to trike by herself."

What. In. The. Actual. Fuck?

I turned the walker around to glare at him. He didn't notice, and I was too stunned to speak. Fuming, I got into my car and slammed the door without another word. I headed to our favorite coffee shop where we had planned to have lunch.

Did he just . . . ? What the . . . ? Every thought ended with a stream of expletives.

I hadn't been so angry since Dad told me the reason he and Mom always asked me out to lunch after swimming. Apparently, they worried I wouldn't eat otherwise. That I wouldn't take the time or was incapable of getting my own food. And here I'd always been plagued by guilt when I begged off lunch to work on Team Drea. I was angry because they didn't want to spend time with me—they just wanted to hover, protect, and *parent* me. *Why did you raise me to be so damn independent if you refuse to let go?* More expletives followed in my brain.

The three of us sat down outside the restaurant. We wiped down every conceivable surface and sanitized our hands per the new COVID protocols. I took a deep breath.

"I know you mean well," I said, looking directly into their eyes. "But I have done seventeen marathons and more than sixty races on my own. If you bought that trike just so you can go with me on all my rides, you can return it now."

"Who said that?" Mom said, directing an accusatory glance at my father. Dad didn't seem to register the problem.

"He did," I said, not about to let either of them off the hook. I tolerated them pacing the pool deck as I swam, Dad counting my laps (loudly), and all manner of other affronts to my waning independence. This was the last straw. Straw. Camel. Back. Broken.

As they stuttered some explanations, I realized that Mom actually wanted the trike for exercise. And she had convinced Dad to make the financial splurge by framing the argument as a life-saving measure for their beloved daughter. *Well, shit.*

I was still annoyed. But I appreciated this masterful stroke of Mom's genius. Clearly derived from fifty-seven years of marital negotiations, she knew how to get what she wanted. I was kinda proud of her.

"Really," Mom said. "We don't expect you to only trike with us."

Before guilt sucked me in or I succumbed to a teenager-y eye roll, I said, "Okay, deal." And I decided to let it go.

Driving home, I decided also to be proud of myself. Before I let my fury and frustration show at the bike shop, I had walked away—okay, maybe *huffed* away—but I had kept the anger to myself. When I did address the issue with my parents, I expressed my thoughts calmly and clearly, and kindly. *Like an actual adult. Good job, Drea.*

Their desire to overprotect me paralleled my desire for independence—a typical parent-child growth pattern. ALS had upended the natural evolution of the relationship between adult-parents and adult-child. Unsure of the future, we had all regressed into what we knew: our original parent-child roles. I needed more help than a forty-year-old adult normally would, so they appeared—ready to parent me like I was still a child. It made sense.

After the flight Mom and I took where the engine blew, our relationship *had* grown. Something about holding hands, silently contemplating life, reconnected us. Some of the ice had thawed away, but we both still had work to do.

⊶⊷

The following Saturday, which should have been the SoCal Marathon, David and I went for a run on a nearby greenway.

About two miles in, David passed me on a steep uphill.

I passed him back as I shot down the other side. I was confident on this trail, since I trained on it often. But I misjudged a sharp curve and skidded on some leaves. I braked hard, jerking the trike back onto the path before I slid off into the ravine. I felt the right wheel lift up. The trike dumped me out, then landed on top of me. My left arm and hand took the brunt of the fall, the pavement ripping a hole in the elbow of my long-sleeved running shirt and scraping the skin off my knuckles.

First thought: *Goddammit, my parents were right.*

Next thought: *I'm never going to be allowed to trike alone again.*

David sprinted up to me, panicked and breathless as he always was when I fell. "Okay, you're okay, it's okay. What did you hit? Oh god, you're bleeding!"

"I'm fine, I'm fine," I reassured him, as I always did. Then checked to see if *fine* was actually true. The road rash was pretty serious, probably requiring stitches. Then reality got really real.

No way can I go to urgent care right now, picturing all the people with COVID. *How could I have been so reckless? What if I had been alone?*

"I'm fine," I said again, firmer this time. I had to be fine. "I'm sorry."

David twisted the heels of my bike shoes, freeing me from the clips on the trike. He righted the trike as I lay on the pavement, helpless.

I had only flipped the trike once before. On one of our first outings, I went barreling down a steep, bowl-shaped hill, aiming for enough speed to make it up to the top on the other side. But like a doomed Looney Tunes character, I *almost* reached the top, remained suspended for a beat too long while my eyes bugged out of my head, then I rolled backward the way I'd come. Panicking, I swerved to the left into the grass and flipped over. David sprinted up, expecting death and destruction, only to find me laughing hysterically with the trike on top of me.

But this time, we weren't laughing.

Neither of us spoke as the rush of adrenaline, fear, and anger subsided from our veins. Silently, he picked the leaves and tiny bits of gravel out of my bloody knuckles and wiped the dirt off with his T-shirt. I refused to flinch.

"Can you make it back to the car?" he asked when I was seated and clipped back into the trike.

I nodded. "I'll be careful," I said.

On the way back, steering with one hand as blood dripped down my arm, I made myself all sorts of promises. I would not go to urgent care and risk getting COVID. Gone was the bravado. I would sit at home, like a good girl, throughout the rest of the pandemic.

There was so much need, so much pain in our country and around the world. But my biggest contribution to society was to stay at home and do nothing. *Be quiet. Be a good girl. Do not be a burden in this current healthcare crisis.*

COVID was, in fact, killing people. In a hauntingly similar way to ALS: suffocation. This was not lost on me. I could hold space for those suffering, dying, and mourning their loved ones.

But righteous indignation swelled up as I read petty complaints about quarantine on social media. People complaining about being told to stay home—to save themselves and their loved ones from a deadly disease. A preventable way to avoid suffocating to death—and yet, people were whining about it. *You feel cooped up in your house? Try being locked inside your body—until you die. I see your quarantine complaints, and I raise you ALS.*

My resentment extended to the world's governments who found untold millions to pump into research to find a cure for COVID. Where was that urgency and money to cure ALS?

Then came the economic assistance programs rolling out to help individuals, families, and businesses impacted by COVID through no fault of their own. Again, I logically understood the need for financial relief. I got it. *I get it. All families affected by ALS get it.*

While private insurance, Medicare, and Medicaid cover the costs of most durable medical equipment, like wheelchairs, that was just the tip of the iceberg when it comes to ALS needs. But outside of these expenses, there is little to no financial assistance for families impacted by ALS. ALS families typically receive the catastrophic diagnosis, followed most often by a sudden loss of income, plus the outrageous cost of caregiving, accessible vehicles, and home renovations required to provide basic accessibility. The list goes on and on.

I had read so many stories about families bankrupted by ALS. Where was the financial relief for us?

For one horrible second, I wished ALS was contagious. (I was definitely not my best self at this moment.)

When the Alaska race was canceled, I allowed myself a small pity party. The documentary was not important in the grand scheme of the current world tapestry of suffering. But it mattered to *me*. Without Alaska, what would the plot of the film be? Woman with terminal illness sets out on impossible marathon quest, only to have it thwarted by a global pandemic, the end?

I had accepted that ALS might prevent my ability to keep doing marathons. A hard outcome, sure, but at least the film would bring awareness. But a global pandemic? Months (years?) could pass before races started up again. Who knew what my health would be like in months or years? I was already living on borrowed time.

I was stuck indefinitely at #17, wondering if I had made a huge mistake investing so much of our foundation's resources into a film about marathons—when all the marathons had vanished.

None of this anxiety, sadness, or anger was productive. I just didn't know what to do with it.

You can be depressed or you can live your life. The time will pass either way. The words came back to me—the ones I had said to myself sitting in the driveway the day I tripped on the rug at work. I had lived an amazing life, in spite of ALS. But if I wanted to give myself the best possible shot at continuing to live, I needed to maintain my strength—even without swimming and the weird Pilates machines I'd come to know and love.

Which meant getting back on the trike safely—and, in my Andrea way—also finding a goal.

I bought a bike computer to track my mileage. I signed up for ALS TDI's Tri-State Trek—a 270-mile bike ride that takes place over three days in New England. The Trek, like most events, was forced to go virtual in 2020.

The Trek had pumped nearly $10 million into the nonprofit lab over fifteen years. Riders nicknamed the event "Trekmas," a weekend they looked forward to all year. Hundreds of riders bonded over blisters, beers, and memories of their loved ones and those fighting ALS. In non-COVID times, David and I flew to Connecticut in time to meet the Trek riders for Saturday night dinner. As the sun set, riders gathered for an open mic night in which anyone could share a testimonial about their loved one with ALS or what Trek meant to them. Listening to the stories reminded everyone why they rode. On the last day, I rode the last ten miles with the scientists from the lab, an honor I coveted. Even though I had to pedal as hard as I could to keep up with the two-wheel road bikes (and they still had to slow down), I loved riding in the pack.

In 2020, ALS TDI needed support more than ever. The pandemic canceled the Trek, the gala, and hundreds of smaller fundraisers that usually kept the lab running. In lean times previously, the development and administrative staff had taken a temporary pay cut to keep the scientists working. But nothing could overcome a deficit in fundraising of this magnitude.

Since the Trek was virtual this year, I decided to ride all 270 miles on my trainer. That way, I reasoned, I could safely keep my fitness up with the added benefit of watching TV.

But even a reality show junkie like me got bored after about three weeks. I missed riding the trails and marathons. I even missed hills.

David felt cooped up, too, and spent an entire weekend cleaning out and rearranging the garage to hang a speed bag. He started participating in the virtual workouts his boxing coach offered daily. He frequently walked in from the garage dripping with sweat.

"Do you think I can do loops in the cul-de-sac while you're in the garage working out? I'll be careful," I added.

⁂

When we looked for a house in Raleigh, we wanted proximity to a running and biking trail. Quickly, we realized that other features had to take priority: a one-story house with a wide hallway to fit a ginormous wheelchair. Even though I was still using a walker and my own two feet, we had to plan. The line from the ALS Clinic had been drilled into me: you have to stay ahead of the disease.

Most "Raleigh ranches" built in the 1950s–1970s had hallways thirty-six inches wide. Thirty-six inches is a standard width for an ADA-compliant doorway, but it's not very comfortable to navigate for the length of a hallway. My wheelchair (already acquired to stay ahead of the disease) was thirty inches wide, leaving only three inches on either side to spare. In addition, Raleigh ranches tend to have small bathrooms, which won't work with a ginormous wheelchair, a caregiver, and potentially a Hoyer lift.

I never envisioned choosing a home based on stair count, hallway width, threshold transitions, maneuverability around kitchen islands, and the size of the bathrooms. But those factors *always* became the dealbreakers.

After a year of house hunting, Mom-the-Realtor spotted a midcentury modern ranch. It had a garage to accommodate a platform lift, space to add on an accessible bathroom, and a hallway with linen closets on either side that could be removed. David and I jumped at it—and high. We offered thirty thousand dollars over the asking price. I wrote an impassioned letter to the seller about how I would love nothing more than to spend my remaining days in their beautiful home.

Nine months and a six-figure renovation later, we had our fully accessible home on a suburban cul-de-sac.

And with that, my fall from urban planner grace was complete.

⊸⧽⧼⊷

To log my miles for the Trek, I pedaled in circles around our tiny cul-de-sac.

My friend Glynis called my circles "Hamster Time." Actually, the route my bike computer plotted was more like a drawing of a lollipop scribbled by some sort of deranged toddler. We lived at the bottom of a small hill, so that was decent hill training. *Up, up, up* I went toward the main road, U-turn, and then flew back down the hill, loop around the bulb of the cul-de-sac, then start the tenth-of-a-mile trek up again.

The cul-de-sac hill was more challenging than the constant flatness of the trainer. With the challenge of it, I felt my spunk coming back. Fresh air combined with budding flowers and trees, breaking into a sweat, feeling my muscles strain against the hill, I remembered myself and how far I had come.

In mid-May, I wrote about my disappointment in missing the Alaska marathon:

> *Tomorrow is not promised; it never was.*
>
> *My brain is exhausted. That feels like post-diagnosis too . . . when the shock of learning I was going to die soon stunned my brain into silence.*
>
> *In the silence, my heart stepped forward.*
>
> *The heart didn't command the lead, the way my brain would, asserting its power over everything. Instead, it whispered . . .* What matters most now? What will bring you joy? How can you make the world better?
>
> *Now I have six years of beautiful memories, a flock of swallow tattoos on my arm, and a community of friends who have stepped up over and over again to support me, us, and ALS research.*
>
> *Races will come back; the documentary will be finished.*
>
> *I will remain strong enough for another thirty-three marathons. If nothing else, the past six years have taught me patience.*

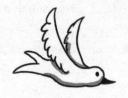

CHAPTER 30

MOTHER'S DAY

May 2020

Mother's Day 2020 created a lot of angst in our house.

I had the mother-child relationship on one hand, then me, childless, on the other. Between quarantine and my race goals being quashed, Mother's Day just added a layer to the gloom. But the truth? The mother stuff—all of it—had been weighing me down for a while. I was tired of carrying it.

I could also tell that David was not okay. I sensed he was carrying a heaviness. I had to do something about it.

First, I wrote Mom a letter. I gave it to her in the driveway, as we sat outside to enjoy a socially distanced picnic.

"You can read it later," I said.

> *Dear Mom,*
>
> *I just wanted to take a little more space than a card to express how very much you mean to me. I really miss our swim sessions, lunches, and trips to Pilates. Getting to spend time with you and Dad is the reason we moved back to NC and I am thankful every day that we made that decision . . .*

I want you to know that especially because I'm not always good at telling you. I roll my eyes, dismiss your suggestions, and bristle each time you over-help, not knowing where that ever-moving line is.

Leading up to my 40th year, I am finally trying to grow out of my teenage angst. And I'd like your help.

I am learning to forgive myself for my major failures: the time I refused to talk to you on your birthday, all the battles leading up to the wedding, and the myriad of times and ways I have been dismissive or rude over the years.

You were, are, and always have been, an incredible mom. You always tried to put my well-being, happiness, and needs first. You always tried your absolute hardest to be there for me and to celebrate my accomplishments, even when I pushed you away.

I would like to move forward as adult friends who also share a tight mother-daughter bond. You will only ever have one daughter, and I will only ever have one mother, so let's celebrate that.

I love you so much and all the years we have to look forward to together!

Love always,

Andrea

No apology in the letter. I had apologized so many times. And Mom already forgave me; I knew she did because she is that kind of person.

This letter was about forgiving *myself*. Saying what I needed to say so that I could move forward and live without the guilt. *Truly live, not just not die.*

It seemed to work—for both of us.

I felt physically lighter after giving her the letter. When COVID protocols eased so we could return to the pool, our relationship had changed. Mom wasn't so afraid of doing the wrong thing; I wasn't so afraid of snapping at her. I no longer had to filter the thoughts in my head so only kind words came out. The inner dialogue was quiet.

⁂

On to David. Although he rallied and acted normal sitting with my parents in the driveway, the rest of the day he was quiet—too quiet. *Uh-oh.*

When I tried to inquire, I got shut down with one-word answers and clipped responses. But I knew. It was *Mother's* Day.

He'd recently brought up trying to have a baby again.

"What if—well, I was just thinking—since you're so stable . . ." he started, haltingly.

The conversation did not go well. I was completely caught off guard and unprepared. So, in my nervousness, I rattled off a list of every practical issue we'd have to figure out and all the hurdles we'd have to overcome.

Pregnancy was hard on any woman's body, so who knew what would happen to mine? We'd discussed surrogacy in the past, but how would we manage an infant? And I would probably still die in the next few years—so even if we worked out all the caregiving complications, wouldn't my death devastate the child? How could we bring a child into the world *knowing* they'd have to lose their mother?

One look at David's face told me that I'd taken the wrong approach.

"Just forget it," he'd said, turning away from me. "I'm not having a baby with someone who doesn't want to." And walked out of the room.

Dammit. His words stung. But I understood. I could tell how hurt he was, realizing that my decision was closing a door. A door he thought might have been cracked open again.

I sat quietly for a long time. *He's not wrong.* I realized that I didn't want to have a baby—not like this. Up until that time, I hadn't had the courage to admit it, even to myself.

We went to bed silently.

David usually falls asleep in three breaths, so I figured I could wait him out. I lay on my side of the bed, frozen, scarcely breathing. A fat tear rolled down my cheek. *Dammit. Just wait a little longer.*

Then came my telltale giveaway—I sniffled. *Dammit!*

David exhaled. "What's wrong?"

"Nothing," I tried to say, but the word came out as a massive, unrecognizable sob. That opened the floodgates.

"Oh, babe," he said. *Dammit.* He rolled toward me and pulled me close. But I didn't want him to comfort me. *Anything* but that. At this point, his loving kindness just drove the dagger further into my gut. I preferred the silent treatment—at least I could stay mad at him for that.

I cried shaking sobs for a long time, as David stroked my hair.

"Can you tell me what you're crying about?" he asked. A ridiculous question. He knew, just like I'd known all day. I shook my head.

"Can you type it on your phone?" Our standard workaround when I was too upset to talk. We'd even had fights through the Notes app.

I didn't want to say what I was thinking this time, but I was too miserable to care anymore.

I typed: "I wish I'd died so you could have had children with someone else." And then I cried even harder.

The next day, I wrote the letter I should have written long before. In four pages of painstakingly chosen words, I explained what I thought our options were.

The first option was having a baby. With that, I pictured Liam, the toddler from the ob-gyn's office who tried to run away with my walker. I wrote how I could not care for a baby, toddler, or young child alone because I could not ensure their safety:

> *All the while knowing I probably wouldn't live to see the child grow up. The sadness almost rips me apart just thinking about it, so I can't imagine the reality.*
>
> *So, we would need a live-in nanny (and nighttime help?) and everything else would fall to you. A nanny we would want to live with and trusted completely. Essentially, you and the nanny would be raising the child because I could not be trusted on my own.*
>
> *I do not want to raise a child like that. I am so, so, so sorry.*

The second option was adoption or fostering an older child. An unfathomable long shot.

My research had revealed that no domestic agency or foreign government allows adoption by a terminally ill parent. I understood the reasoning behind this protection for a child. But also . . . *what?* There wasn't a child anywhere in the world I was fit to parent, no matter how much of a loving home we could offer? That realization dragged me into such a pit of despair and unworthiness that I could not even look at it head-on. I gave up immediately. I could not bear to pile on the heartbreak or expense of pursuing adoption.

The final option gutted me. It was the hardest, saddest option of all. I offered to set David free.

> *You would be an amazing dad and I HATE that I am standing in the way of that. Couples break up because one person wants kids and one doesn't.*
>
> *Our situation is not the same, but the outcome is.*
>
> *This isn't about "fighting for our marriage" or "making it work."*
>
> *It isn't about not loving you enough—it's the exact opposite. I'm offering this precisely because that is how much I love you.*
>
> *I have had an amazing life because of you. I want you to have an amazing life too.*
>
> *I am not ready to die, but I don't want you to live a life you don't want because of me. I am very serious about this. I will never hold it against you.*

I meant every word.

The only other option was us. Just as we were and would be.

Childless. The one option where Mother's Day and Father's Day would always be hard. This was the option I wanted—but only if David did too.

I wrote that I could handle anything he had to say, any decision he made. I meant that, too.

So, not knowing what was left to do, I thrust the letter into David's hands as he was leaving to run errands. I wanted him to have time—alone—to process his thoughts.

"Here," I said. "This will be hard to read, so wait until you're ready. I love you."

He looked at me quizzically.

"Just trust me," I said. He nodded.

When he closed the door, I waited for the tears to come. After all, I might have just thrown away my marriage, my soulmate, and my life as I knew it.

I felt dizzy. I pushed my walker over to the couch and sat down shakily. My heart was beating fast, but a calmness began to take hold deep inside of me. The tears didn't come.

I was honest with him—and *finally*—with myself. That calmed me.

Yes, I wanted to be a mother. I wanted to have a child. *Before.*

But ALS changed that, like it had changed every other part of me. Living with ALS was now my reality. And I couldn't reconcile motherhood and ALS.

I refused to feel guilty about it any longer.

∞

David was gone for a long time.

I was feeding the cats when he walked in the door. He walked straight over to me and wrapped his arms around me. We stood that way for what felt like an eternity, neither of us wanting to let go.

When we finally pulled apart, he cupped my face in his hands in the way that I love.

"I choose you" is all he said. That's all I needed to hear.

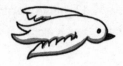

CHAPTER 31

BUY THE DAMN BOAT

August 2020

"BUY THE DAMN BOAT," reads the sign on our newly added-on screened-in porch.

The quote is from William "Cory" Burell, a friend who died of ALS in 2019, just five days before his thirty-sixth birthday. When David and I met Cory and his wife, Alison, we became inseparable.

Cory knew ALS all too well. His father died from it when Cory was thirteen.

"I made it a point after losing my father to ALS to never take my foot off the gas," Cory wrote in a long social media post (manifesto, really) three years after his diagnosis. The post was unusual in its length—but also unusual in its absence of snark. Cory had spectacular snark.

For example, immediately after his trach surgery, Cory decided to let us know he had survived the surgery and (bonus!) could still speak a little in a gravelly voice. So, he recorded and sent us the following voice memo: *Fuuuuuck the Eagles. Fuuuuck them in the ass. Love you, David.* Click.

The Eagles are David's favorite team.

Cory's social media manifesto read:

I kept death in the back of my mind [which has] both hurt and
helped me. . . .

Take whatever task is in front of you and destroy it with your
willpower. Don't accept what anyone tells you your limitations are. . . .

Make all your mistakes, don't let them slow you down—let them
make you a better person. Dive deep into your soul and ask yourself
what your purpose is and what you should be doing. Don't be afraid
to address your mortality, your current life, and your faith, or you will
never truly live. . . . Never die wishing you had grabbed an experience
in life, made a difference in the world, or lived it differently. Nothing
is guaranteed so be who you want to be now.

Oh, and for God's sake, just buy the damn boat if you want it.

The screened-in porch was my damn boat.

If I progressed to the point that I could no longer leave the house, I reasoned, I could live out my remaining days happily sweating on the porch. I
am one of those annoying people who enjoys humidity. So why not go ahead
and build the damn porch?

We built the porch in the fall of 2019, which turned out to be perfect
timing. I spent the summer of quarantine on the porch writing and reading.
I obsessively checked marathon schedules. Every single race was canceled
or postponed indefinitely. The running industry was another casualty of
COVID.

But wait . . . what's this?

Idaho, Wyoming, Utah: Marathons #18, #19, and #20

The Bear Lake Marathon Trifecta: Idaho, Wyoming, and Utah. Three races
in three states in three days. Three weeks out. "Only" 2,148 miles away.

"David!" I called in the direction of the adjacent home office where he had
been working full-time. "You want to drive to Idaho with me in three weeks
to race?"

He came out, eyes wide. "You want to drive all the way to Idaho to do a marathon?"

I shook my head and held up three fingers. *Three.* I grinned.

Why not? We had no kids to homeschool. David hadn't taken a day off all year. We, like most everyone, had been cooped up at home for four months.

Am I a hypocrite—going to do something like this? Probably. Yes, I had cringed watching the videos of pandemic parties in Florida. But we weren't going to do *that.* Masks, hand sanitizer, disinfecting wipes, not eating in restaurants—we knew the protocols. Besides, my life was on borrowed time. I was six years into a terminal illness with an average life expectancy of two to five years. Who knew how long my body could finish marathons?

My left knee still threatened to give out. After 270 miles in the cul-de-sac, it now hurt with every ride. Mischa and I had been working to strengthen it, but then COVID shut everything down. We tried Zoom sessions, using whatever props I had on hand: a chair, a magic circle, resistance bands. It was something, but not nearly as effective as the Pilates studio equipment.

A knee brace helped, as did ice packs after training and stretching. Could my knee hold up through thirty-three more marathons? No idea. But three marathons in three days was a good start and a big test. I had to try.

❦

Bear Lake boasted itself as the "Caribbean of the Rockies" on its website. I was skeptical. That sort of advertising felt like the local Chamber of Commerce got carried away. I was wrong.

After three days in the car, David and I arrived at a stunning turquoise lake. Indeed, bluer than the Caribbean. The color is due to limestone deposits suspended in the water. The Chamber of Commerce actually undersold this place. Mountains framed the lake with a wide sandy beach ringing the shoreline. Umbrellas out. People, but plenty of social distance.

I turned to David with a pleading look. "Beach day tomorrow?"

He laughed. "Sure thing."

The next morning, we paid a park fee and then drove *right up onto* the beach. As a Carolina girl, driving on any beach felt like sacrilege. But this was allowed. The beach had no dunes to protect—just hard-packed sand—and a stunning, panoramic view of blue sky, blue lake, and gray-blue mountains.

We picked a spot away from others. My walker doesn't roll on sand, so we left it behind. David steadied me, walking backward toward the water, holding both of my hands in his. Talk about romantic. We yelped a little as the frigid water gently washed over our feet.

But here, with no tides, no crashing waves, no undertow threatening to pull me under—*I can swim!* But first we had to get deep enough in the water.

Backward and forward we walked. Even after ten minutes, the crystal-clear water had only reached our knees. I stopped, taking in the breathtaking landscape.

David stood behind me, his arms around my waist. I leaned back, secure against his chest. I couldn't give him a child, but I could give him a lifetime of adventures—including this spectacular corner of the world. He chose me, just like I chose him. All those years ago and every day since.

Staring out at the blue everything, I wondered once again about how much beauty *is* in the breakdown, the destruction of current life—the way things must sometimes fade and die, in order to regrow and thrive.

⤜⤛

The Bear Lake Trifecta avoided a crowd by having a ninety-minute rolling-start window. That meant no pre-race panic about oversleeping, getting dressed, forgetting something, cramming in breakfast, getting lost on the way to the start, parking, pumping tires, setting GoPros, tightening knee braces—any and all of which had threatened my start in past races. These races? My time started whenever I, well, *started*.

Idaho (#18) was up first in the trifecta. I cruised up and down the hills of Bear Lake. I looked out over the lake almost the entire race. It was hard to look away. I had déjà vu. But from where? *Oh!* The Maui Marathon. Mountain or volcano on one side, sparkling water on the other. Hawaii and Idaho—never would have compared the two.

Wyoming (#19) was nothing like Idaho or Hawaii. I pedaled 13.1 miles out, turned around, and went back the same way. My view was miles of dry, brown soil studded with tufts of hearty grasses, sunburned scrub bushes, and the occasional cow. *Moo.*

Even in the absence of extraordinary beauty, I felt extraordinary life in Wyoming.

I scarcely looked at the miles or my pace. I did not push for time. I pushed for experience, for life, for *this right now* adventure. The gift of being alive (and healthy) was never more present than right there on my trike in Wyoming.

Lucky. The word resounded in my head.

I used to believe that everything happened for a reason. Like my ALS diagnosis, plus the number 179 connection to Jon Blais that led to my "last race," which subsequently led to creating the Team Drea Foundation, was all predestined to mean something. Some grand plan. Some grand *why*, that could somehow justify all the pain.

I didn't believe that anymore.

Things certainly *happen*, but it's up to us, individually, to give that thing a *reason*. To lend our perspective. To make something meaningful out of tragedy. To help others in ways that we can, and they cannot. This is how we express our appreciation for the gifts we have. This is what makes us *human*.

I would call myself spiritual, but not religious. I'm agnostic in my belief about an afterlife* beyond the specks of life begetting new life. How we spend our time and whatever we create lives on, but these are the only moments we are promised. And that's what makes them precious.

Lucky is my best explanation for being born in America to wonderful parents who raised me to work hard. *Lucky* to have met and loved and married David—my person, the one who makes me better than I am. The only *unlucky* thing was ALS, and I seem to have won the damn ALS lottery.

Oh, the guilt I have carried about my slow ALS progression.

Cory, sarcasm and all, would have given anything to watch his boys grow into men. Yet, his fervent desire to live could not overpower the relentless progression of his disease. The disease that extinguished one body part at a time.

---

* However, Cory's memorial service made me think twice about proof of an afterlife. As soon as the service began, the lights flickered. They stopped after a minute or two, but started up again when his wife, Alison, spoke. Cory had worked in the electrical construction industry for fifteen years. Honestly, a light show is exactly the kind of shit he would pull at his own funeral.

But my feeling guilty doesn't do a thing for Cory. Not now, nor when he was alive.

Guilt could not and will not save anyone from anything—ALS or COVID or cancer, or any other tragedy. Guilt doesn't do anything for anyone.

I was tired of guilt. It had taken up too much of my life already.

Instead of guilt over my slow ALS progression, I would honor my friends by spending my remaining time in the bravest, most joyful, purpose-filled way I could find.

I looked out at the otherworldly Wyoming landscape and lonely ribbon of highway I'd never see again but would forever remember.

Guilt is a waste of time and emotion. I choose to be brave.

⁂

To Utah (#20), I brought a left knee that was super twingey at the start line. It *was* the third day in a row of 26.2 miles. I was tired.

David crouched down to slip the GoPro cameras onto the trike. Seconds after he turned the cameras on, I let out a huge fart.

"Huh," David said. "Loud geese today."

I laughed so hard that I farted again. Well, *that* opened the floodgates—both in laughter and sphincter. I spent the first mile fart-giggling, and it brought me the joy and energy I needed for the last day of racing—which I knew would be the hardest yet. Difficult indeed, but new momentum had ignited. The Bear Lake Trifecta was just what I needed to get back on the road again.

⁂

On the drive back home, I received a text from my Team Drea board member Ashley.

Gauging from the excessive emojis, she was excited. *She's probably pregnant again.* She and her husband, Doug, already had four kiddos to chase around the DC suburbs.

"And no, I'm not pregnant again" came the next text.

"Call me!" she said, with more excited emojis.

In DC, Ashley and I had lived only fifteen minutes apart, so we started running together. We did my first half marathon together, after I realized ALS wasn't ravaging my body as quickly as expected.

Ashley had been a serious runner since college—sprinter, actually. At her first 5K with Team Drea in 2015, she won! She broke the tape of the Miami Marathon 5K with a blazing fast speed of 6:04 per mile. She also won the Cherry Blossom 5K that year.

But in August 2018, I received a text from Doug: "Andrea, Ashley is OK, but she got hit by an SUV in a crosswalk while running this morning."

My heart stopped, right as my phone rang. It was Doug.

"Oh my god! Is she okay?"

"She's okay. She has a fractured left ankle and broken right wrist . . . but she's okay." He reassured us. *Wait, opposite ankle and wrist?*

Ashley had been running in a well-marked crosswalk when she looked up to see a large SUV barreling toward her. Instinctively, she put her right arm out. When the vehicle hit her wrist, her body fell forward and slammed into the ground. The SUV ran over both her legs, fracturing her left ankle.

My hand flew up to my mouth.

"We are just so grateful it wasn't worse. And that she wasn't running and pushing the kids in the stroller." *Oh my god, yes.*

How could Doug be so calm? My fury at the driver exploded. She was in a *crosswalk*, she was a *mother*, and she was my *dear friend*. She wasn't just a recreational runner, she *won* races! Now, would she ever run again?

She and Doug had been part of Team Drea since the beginning. They were both board members. I couldn't imagine Ashley, of all people, *not* being okay.

Much to my relief, when I visited a few weeks later, Ashley was hopping around on one foot, pushing her modified walker with a cradle for her bandaged wrist. *What amazing motor neurons you have, my dear!*

"I think of you all the time these days," she said, plopping onto the couch. She somehow wrapped her good arm around her youngest child and hoisted him onto her lap to nurse.

"I don't see how you do it," she said. *Right back at you, Ashley.*

So, the text from Ashley I received in Wyoming said to call immediately. She answered breathless, which I figured was from chasing kids, but no—it was the excitement reflected in her text.

"You know, the accident," she started. "We never knew if we would get a settlement, but we wanted to try. We just wanted the driver held accountable."

Crash! Commotion in the background. Little kid voices squabbling.

"Doug! Can you get . . .? Hang on, sorry," Ashley said. I grinned. Our conversations always went like this.

"Anyway, Doug and I said that if we ever got a settlement for pain and suffering, like after the medical bills were paid, we would give it to Team Drea for the film."

She paused. My eyes widened.

She continued, her voice rising with excitement, "Andrea, it's $45,000!"

I almost dropped the phone.

Our business plan for the documentary never quite yielded major corporate sponsors, though not for lack of trying. I guess it was hard to believe I would live to see fifty marathons. Catrike made a wonderful donation, as did our local Subaru dealership and Rotary Club.

In the void, Team Drea board members individually stepped in and donated the majority of funds needed for the original vision to produce the fifty-minute short film through Alaska at #21. When COVID hit, we'd agreed to keep filming on the GoPros, hoping something would work out.

And now, it had. Ashley's donation would almost fully fund the remaining production costs for a *full-feature film with fifty marathons*.

Sputtering, I did my best to thank Ashley and Doug for their generosity. As always with heartfelt donations, I felt my words were woefully inadequate to convey my gratitude. How do you thank someone for believing in you? For helping you fulfill your life's purpose?

Some people, it turns out, don't buy the boat. They pay it forward instead.

CHAPTER 32

FALLING APART

Indiana, Illinois, Kansas, and Missouri:
Marathons #21, #22, #23, and #24
September–November 2020

Now that we had broken the seal on travel, it was open season. No state in America was safe—well, except the ones where I had done marathons already.

A month after our almost-cross-country trek to Bear Lake, I persuaded David to take a weekend jaunt to the Fair on the Square Marathon in Indiana (#21), one of only six in-person marathons in the country that weekend.

A few weeks later, Shaw and I took a road trip to hit the Dam Site Run (#22) in southern Illinois, then the Little Apple Marathon (#23) in Manhattan, Kansas, and finally, the Bass Pro Conservation Marathon (#24) in Springfield, Missouri.

In between marathon weekends, Shaw and I holed up in a quarantine-type vacation rental in Kansas City for a glorious workcation. During our trip, I realized how drastically my own speaking patterns had been forced to change. In conversations with Shaw, a self-proclaimed extreme extrovert, I had to plan each anecdote carefully: mentally shortening phrases before I spoke them, steering clear of three- and four-syllable words. Incredibly frustrating. I couldn't carry on a normal girls' trip conversation, spiked with homemade cocktails and general silliness.

My left knee was also becoming increasingly painful during the fall races. But these things were only annoyances. I remembered how *lucky* I was not to have to use eye gaze or a phone to read my words. How lucky I was to have the strength and the motor neuron connections to pedal.

Control what you can control, I soothed myself whenever anxiety threatened to overwhelm my perspective. *ALS could be so very much worse.*

Florida: Marathon #25
December 2020

Looking at my wall map, the only remaining state likely to have a marathon in December within driving distance was Florida.

"It's only seven hours away!" I wheedled when I found the Sandy Claus Run near Jacksonville.

"Andrea, no. It's *Florida*," David said, having watched the same news coverage I had with crowded beaches, packed bars, and COVID cases spiking.

But I also wanted to go to Florida because the awesome folks at Catrike (located in Orlando) were giving me a new folding trike, plus a bag to carry it in. Dad would no longer have to bubble wrap the trike! I wanted to pick up the trike and thank Catrike in person.

The debate went on for days. Eventually, David reluctantly agreed, so I registered before he could change his mind.

Four days before our planned Florida departure, I bent down to rummage through a bottom drawer and felt a pop in my back. I tried to stand up. The pain took my breath away.

David was running errands, so I pushed my walker back to the couch, completely bent over at the waist. In that position, I felt okay. *Maybe I can straighten . . .? Nope, no, I can't.* Stars appeared before my eyes. I almost passed out from the pain.

I had heard people say "I threw my back out," but never understood. *Oh boy, now I do.*

After lying on my back for two days on a heating pad, my muscles relaxed a little. David, to his immense credit given the tension between us over Florida, stepped up caregiving without complaint—food, ibuprofen, readjusting pillows, lifting me in and out of the bed. *This is what life with ALS is like for most people. I cannot imagine.*

But I could. I had been picturing this life for almost seven years. Maybe David had as well.

With hours of uninterrupted thinking time, I reconsidered—everything. Confronted with a glimpse of our very likely future, Florida was both less and more important. The exact race was *less* important, but the fifty-marathon challenge was *more* important.

My body had to decide. Well, and David too. Through a heartfelt apology and a long discussion, we agreed to make the trip as long as I honored my body's needs.

I hoped I could be honest with myself.

I showed up at the start line in Nocatee, Florida, and within no time, I was in darkness.

"It is so dark," I gasped. "Jesus!"

Next to me, Brian was running full speed, trying to hold his camera steady.

We were hurtling through pitch-black darkness on a trail through a swamp. No wonder the race director had strapped a bike light to the front of the trike, though it wasn't illuminating much more than my white bike shoes passing each other. I had worried about COVID, my back, and my knee—but not alligators, snakes, or god knows what other creatures out here before the sun rose.

Nocatee is one of those massive master planned communities I'd studied in planning school. With twenty-two neighborhoods covering 15,000 acres, Nocatee incorporated all the services residents needed to live, work, and play without ever leaving. Now, in the darkness of the swamp, I wondered if we were about to encounter the same fate.

My back was stiffening up, and my left knee throbbed.

By the time I crossed the line at the slow time of 4:18:26, I couldn't believe my exhaustion from such a flat course. *COVID? ALS progression? My back? Twelve races in one year? Who knew.*

Then my exhaustion lifted and my heart lit up when I realized something: *I'm halfway done with FIFTY marathons. Hot damn!*

CHAPTER 33

21 IN '21

I had always imagined Boston as my fiftieth marathon, and something about hitting the halfway mark stoked the fire even more. But I still wasn't sure if the BAA would allow me to participate.

On the other hand, the Prince of Wales Island Marathon had already welcomed me with open arms. Originally scheduled as #21 for May 2020, thanks to COVID, the race had a new date of May 2022. The race organizers remained excited about *me* as their guest speaker, but now, after two years of talking about it, the whole *island* seemed excited about *all* of Team Drea coming. Enthusiastic social posts and a steady stream of emails from locals, athletes, and businesses let us know how much everyone on the island looked forward to our arrival.

Originally, Alaska was to be the finale of the short-film documentary.

But what if Alaska was the finale of a *full-length* documentary? *And* Marathon #50?

That would give me eighteen months to complete twenty-four more marathons. Eighteen months without getting injured or sick, without the airlines damaging the trike, without any other mishaps forcing a missed race. Seemed crazy, but what in this journey hadn't been?

I emailed dozens of race officials, explaining my quest and asking if I could participate in their marathons. More races began saying yes—maybe because

I'd already completed so many? Maybe it was the prospect of being featured in a documentary? Either way, my race calendar began filling up, fast.

Maryland and Rhode Island: Marathons #26 and #27
April 2021

After a four-month break to rehab my knee, David and I drove to Maryland for the weekend and checked off #26 with the Salisbury Marathon.

Next, Jillaine and I drove to Newport, Rhode Island, for #27. This particular trip remains locked in infamy forever—not only because of the race, but because of the time Jillaine *ran over my walker* with the car . . . because I told her to.

"It's stuck or something," Jillaine had said, after she slid into the driver's seat to drive my car for the first time.

"Just give it a little more gas," I coaxed. "It's fine." The car lurched forward, then smoothed out.

"Oh shit. Your walker!" she said, looking in the rearview mirror.

Whoops. I was so accustomed to David putting the walker in the car that I hadn't thought to mention it to Jillaine. Neither of us had done it. So when I told her to give it gas—I encouraged her to actually run over my walker. *Have mercy.*

As Jillaine circled back to retrieve it, I could see from the passenger seat that we had a problem.

"Oh well, it's fine. It'll still hold me up," I said, looking at a now-non-turning wheel.

"No way." Jillaine bought me a new walker—that day.

With a spike in COVID cases over the winter, the in-person race had been rescheduled once again for a later date. Since Jillaine and I along with her sister, Jodi, had already made our plans and the filmmakers were joining us, we decided to tackle the course using the race's virtual option.

Jillaine and Jodi lost their mom, Dawn, to ALS in 2009. She had lived less than a year post-diagnosis. The sisters ran the Chicago Marathon to honor the fifth anniversary of their mom's passing. When Jillaine read my story of the Ramblin' Rose triathlon in *Endurance* magazine, she reached out personally to me. Now, I could not imagine life without them.

Jodi surprised us race morning with homemade bibs—all numbered 179—because Rhode Island was Jon Blais's home state. With no official race start time and near-freezing temps, Jillaine, Jodi, and I took our sweet time leaving the cozy rental house.

I spent countless hours plotting the race route in the days leading up to the trip. I mostly adhered to the actual marathon course, but also was forced to adapt for safety conditions to avoid roads open to traffic. I created a course that was part actual race route and part other streets but still covered the magical distance of 26.2 miles.

One critical variable I had forgotten to consider in my course creation, though: elevation change. *Whoops.*

So as the three of us climbed yet another monstrous hill of my own making, the cold and fatigue settled into my bones. *Well, at least we're together.* The bond between us grew stronger with each passing mile. The sisters have said they feel closest to their mom when they run and race, so I pictured Dawn and Jon Blais protecting us as we battled the hills and the elements.

Rain poured on us throughout the back half of the marathon; on aptly named Purgatory Road, the rain pelted us sideways. The ocean was angry; dark, choppy waves tossed spray into the air. *At least we're together.* We turned around at Sachuest Point and confronted the same wind and rain gauntlet on the way back, now assaulting the other side of our faces. Water squished inside my bike shoes.

The race ended unceremoniously when we reached my car. Jodi surprised us again—this time with recycled finisher medals. Her crafty new inscription? *COVID. Race canceled. Finished anyway.*

⁂

Spreading ashes is a tricky business.

When I emptied the small bag of Jon's ashes at the Team Drea party in North Carolina in 2015, I later discovered some of the ashes remained in the bag.

Unsure what to do, I simply put the bag in my nightstand, where it had stayed—for six years.

But when Rhode Island made it on the calendar, I decided to bring part of Jon back home.

At sunset, after we were rested and thawed out from the marathon, Jillaine, Jodi, and I returned to the beach. The low clouds remained, but no longer threatened rain. The ocean had calmed, and so had we.

With a sister on either side holding me up, we walked out to the water's edge. (Even a new walker won't roll on sand.)

Jillaine read Jon's poem. I sobbed. The moment was all too sad, and too beautiful, to do anything else.

> *Understand that this is not a dress rehearsal.*
> *That this is it . . . your life.*
> *Face your fears and live your dreams.*
> *Take it in.*
> *Yes, every chance you get.*
> *Come close,*

(I started laughing—knowing the next line that was coming—as the documentary cameras rolled.)

> *And, by all means, whatever you do*
> *Get it on film.*

Check. I hope we did you proud, Jon. Scratch that. I know we did.

Washington and Oregon: Marathons #28 and #29
May 2021

Clearly, the wildlife was in charge in the Pacific Northwest.

At the Windermere Marathon (#28) outside Spokane, Washington, MJ sent the camera drone into the air—only to have it swarmed by over a hundred barn swallows. *Swallows.* Of all the birds. She tried again. Same thing. Swooping, divebombing swallows—their split tails so distinctive, they couldn't be anything else.

"They're supposed to be on *our* side," MJ said, laughing.

Before leaving Spokane, Elizabeth (back for another college-roommate vacation) and I stopped for my next swallow tattoo.

Swallow tattoo seven was hand-drawn by Ella, Ashley's almost-seven-year-old daughter. I was having a seventh birthday too, in a way. Ella was born around the same time I was diagnosed with probable ALS. Her drawing depicted a swallow with its wings tight against its body—that split tail brilliantly distinctive—looking exactly like a divebombing swallow.

After a weeklong road trip, we arrived in Salem, Oregon, for the Willamette Valley Marathon (#29), where the wildlife continued to rule. The racecourse was rerouted because of a bald eagle nest; then, a family of beavers dammed up the creek and flooded the trail.

Which seemed like the most Oregon problem ever.

In response to the beavers, the race organizers bushhogged a detour and removed stumps for a two-loop marathon course. Like riding a bucking bronco, I bounced along the rutted dirt path hastily cut through the tall grass. Despite my efforts, I found myself stuck on the obstacle course of tree roots. My friend Anna Katherine had to push me through. *Dammit.* I hated accepting help during marathons these days.

For the second loop, in order to avoid the roots, I triked back and forth on the section before the flooded stretch, relying on my bike computer for the mileage.

This is not cheating, I told myself firmly. *Am I in Oregon? Triking 26.2 miles?* Yes and yes.

No guilt. Not gonna let it seep in. Andrea, you are doing it. This is LIVING.

Montana: Marathon #30
Memorial Day Weekend, 2021

The only friend I knew in Montana, Michel, insisted that we stay with her for the weekend, even though we hadn't seen each other since high school. The free lodging plus the $5 entry fee to the Frank Newman Memorial Marathon (#30) (which included a sandwich at the end, courtesy of the Newman family), made Montana the least expensive marathon to date.

I couldn't find an elevation profile for the race, but given that it was *Montana*, I was worried. My only insight: the website advertised an "uphill half" and a "downhill half." The full marathon would do both.

Within the first mile, the entire race left me behind. Not to make it sound too dramatic: there were only five other marathoners and five "uphill half" marathoners, total, but still. I was alone. I deployed every single strategy I knew for grinding up hills on the trike: the weave-back-and-forth-instead-of-trying-to-go-straight-up technique, the brake-pedal-half-a-rotation-brake-reset-feet technique, and—my personal favorite—the make-husband-meet-you-at-the-bottom-of-the-hill-and-walk-up-while-encouraging-you technique.

I never got a helping push, though. My bike computer showed 1,000 feet of uphill climbing in the first seven miles.

While those seven miles took me over two hours to complete, I finished the last *nineteen* in under ninety minutes!

Like a divebombing swallow, I flew. I careened straight down the highway into a valley of green fields, ringed by snow-capped mountains. A big, goofy grin spread across my face and remained there for miles. The glorious spring day, the effort I'd already put in, the joy of being alive—I lived it all on that downhill.

My confidence grew as the miles whizzed by beneath my wheels, down the never-ending hill. The pavement was so good that I let my speedometer creep up. I'd never tested how fast I could go. *Concentrate, concentrate.* One wrong move while bombing down a hill at this speed, well, I just couldn't think about it. *You've got this. Trust yourself.*

Riding just inches above the streaking pavement was thrilling, but I didn't dare look around. My eyes scanned for danger: potholes, debris, glints of glass. I sneaked momentary glances at my speedometer, just to see. *If I reach 30 mph, I quit this crazy divebombing.*

I beamed. *30 mph. There it is.*

For the next year, when anyone asked me about my favorite marathon, Montana was the race I named.

When I saw David and Michel, I almost couldn't speak. Because my smile stretched ear to ear.

"You went *thirty* miles an hour?" David was incredulous. "Don't tell me stuff like that!"

I couldn't help but smile even bigger.

~~Massachusetts~~, Vermont, New Hampshire, Maine, Wisconsin, Minnesota, Nebraska, South Dakota, North Dakota, and New Mexico: Marathons #31, #32, #33, #35, #36, #39, #40, #41, and #45
Mainly Marathons: June–November 2021

Logistically, the only feasible way for me to tackle so many marathons in a year was through the multiday, multistate Mainly Marathons events. The structure of the Mainly Marathons allowed me to knock out several marathons in a row—assuming my body held up.

So, in June, I talked my in-laws into road-tripping around New England to hit four states in a row* with the Loonies and their trademark mascot, the Loon.

First up: Massachusetts. I still hoped for Boston in 2022, but I couldn't hang my fifty-state dream on a race that hadn't allowed me in yet. Mainly Marathons Massachusetts (#31) was my insurance policy.

But now, I had a bigger problem in Massachusetts: one big-ass hill that climbed for a half mile. Because the structure of Mainly Marathons was out and back many times, I would be forced to climb this hill (er, this mini mountain with a steeper incline than the Montana one) *twelve* times. And I still had three more marathons in the following three days.

I could have gotten a push, sure. Every single racer who passed me asked if they could assist. I shook my helmet-head vigorously, knowing my breathy voice wouldn't be audible. Eye contact, shake head, smile.

Thanks to Mischa, my knee was strong. Her Pilates studio was back open. We worked hard to strengthen my glutes, hips, hamstrings, and the muscles around my knee. *But.* I remembered how much pain I was in before, during, and after the Florida marathon. I had promised myself and David to take better care of my health.

I had never—not before ALS and not since—pulled out of a race. The dreaded DNF: did not finish. *Could I really quit?* I turned the thought over

---

* I know what you're thinking—*four* marathons in a row? But hey, I completed three at the Bear Lake Trifecta—what's one more? Besides, the New England series is six states in six days and starts a day after the end of the Independence series, which is five states in five days. There are Loonies who race all eleven days. See? Four marathons in a row doesn't seem so crazy now.

and over in my head. *If I stay in this race, what is the ultimate cost? Am I willing to risk the next three states? Or re-injuring my knee?*

Back down the mini mountain, I told my in-laws I was done for the day. I informed the race directors, brothers Daniel and Jesse, that I'd see them the following day. Before I left, though, I gave a television interview.

Media interviews were a part of Shaw's new marketing plan: to raise awareness (and hopefully, money for ALS) through the local press as I ping-ponged around the country. A committee of Team Drea volunteers researched outlets, sent press releases, and set up interviews. My only job was to answer reporters' questions at the finish line. But a big job for me—to speak after the fatigue of a marathon.

However, the Massachusetts interview was easy, since I hadn't finished the race.

"It just wasn't meant to be," I said to the reporter. "And that's okay. Just live to fight another day. Like tomorrow in Vermont."

⌘

Mainly Marathons Vermont (the new #31) was a much flatter course—much to my relief. And everyone else's.

"Way better than yesterday, huh?" said several Loonies as we passed each other on the back-and-forth course. It rained the entire race, but at least it wasn't cold.

Most of New Hampshire (#32) took place on an unpaved trail, too narrow for the trike to pass. "No problem," Daniel and Jesse had said.

The brothers measured out a modified course on the sidewalk. I just turned right instead of left toward Main Street to see a bit of tiny downtown Claremont, New Hampshire. Jesse ran with me on the first lap to show me where to turn right and where to turn around.

I thanked him for making the race inclusive of people with disabilities.

"We *never* leave anyone behind," Jesse said.

⌘

By Mainly Marathons Maine (#33), I was a bona fide member of the Loony community. We smiled and shouted encouragement at each other like old friends—every single lap. Most of the Loonies *were* longtime friends, meeting up in different corners of the country to walk (running optional), talk, and explore—several times a year. The Loonies carried on long conversations, mostly about races, to pass the miles. They'd walk until mid-afternoon, drive across the next state border, sleep, and do it all again.

There are worse ways to spend a life.

❧

In July, Shaw and I headed to Mainly Marathons Wisconsin (#35), which took place in Sparta: the "Bicycle Capital of America," according to a building-size mural. Sparta boasted the country's first rail-to-trail (abandoned rail line converted to a trail), and its downtown park boasted the World's Largest Bicycling statue. *Ben Bikin'* rode atop a thirty-two-foot penny farthing, the nineteenth-century bicycle with the big front wheel. Roadside Americana at its finest.

I fell comfortably into the rhythm of a Mainly Marathons race: eye contact, smile, shout encouragement. Shaw and I heartily laughed at the "Ewe-Turn" on the course: a cone marking the turnaround, complete with a flock of plastic toy sheep.

After Wisconsin, we headed to St. Cloud, Minnesota. We drank ourselves silly on overpriced cocktails, toasted to friendship, gave two more media interviews, and spent another successful week exploring the Midwest. The next day, I *may* have done Mainly Marathons Minnesota (#36) with a *tiny* hangover, but it was worth it.

❧

In September, at Mainly Marathons Nebraska (#39), Jesse led me out again. The course cut across an off-road section too treacherous for the trike. I loved how much of a non-problem Jesse made any adaptations for me. Almost a shrug. Like, "Of course we can accommodate you." And yet, it meant so much to *me*.

I tried to maintain that gratitude when I discovered my personal detour was one long, evil uphill. I groaned. *I thought Nebraska was flat.*

Doable, though. Just would take a while.

David got bored and went for a hike; I got bored and decided to take advantage of another Mainly perk: the Loony Lunchbox. Forget energy gels and sports drinks, the aid station on the course was a veritable feast for racers: pasta salad, chili, *pancakes*—every loop if you were so inclined. I carefully selected a crispy rice treat and headed back out.

In twelve loops, I climbed 1,100 feet—yep, more than Montana.

At the start of our trip, I had posted a selfie from the airport wheelchair showing David's head floating above mine as he pushed me through the Rapid City airport.

"Who goes to South Dakota for vacation? We do!" read the caption. Only in the days following did I realize how uninformed that statement was. From the Badlands to bison, prairie dogs popping out of holes, and colors in the rocks that shifted as the sun moved—our eyes couldn't absorb the magnificence fast enough.

While the scenery was incredible, I found myself stealing more glances at the sight in the driver's seat.

Twenty years together. I was still giddy to have David all to myself for a whole week. But, of course, we had business to attend to: three marathons in four days.

In contrast to Nebraska, Mainly Marathons South Dakota (#40) and North Dakota (#41) were mercifully flat, perched on the shoulders of drinking water reservoirs. North Dakota displayed such a picturesque sunrise over the lake that I couldn't wait to show the filmmakers my GoPro footage.

On the plane home, I pulled up my helmet cam footage on the computer—only to discover a completely black screen, except for one sliver of blue sky. *Wait, what?* In the dark, we must have put the GoPro in backward. *D'oh.* At least I had the memory.

Finally, in November, Shaw and I took one more weekend adventure to Mainly Marathons New Mexico (#45). I convinced MJ to come because I wanted the documentary to include my Loony friends. *Look! It doesn't matter how old you are. You too can do this!*

Daniel said that some of the Mainly racers are too slow to participate in traditional races. So that was part of the reason behind Mainly Marathons—to include everyone who wanted to race.

"We'll stay out here as long as they do," he said. "So they can keep doing what they love."

This touched me so deeply my heart ached.

Michigan: Marathon #34
June 2021

David and I spent our twelfth wedding anniversary at the MISH Waterfront Marathon (#34) in Michigan. We clinked glasses in the hotel restaurant, overlooking Lake Michigan.

But our thoughts quietly drifted back home.

The unspoken sadness between us came from missing the Celebration of Life for yet another friend, killed off too soon by ALS.

Dr. Michael Bereman had a beautiful life. He was a tenured professor at his alma mater, NC State, and married to the love of his life, Meagan. He loved being a dad to his children, Mason and Millie.

Then his bicep started twitching.

Michael was diagnosed with ALS three days before his thirty-fourth birthday. But he didn't retire. With a PhD in applied chemistry, postdoctoral work in disease biomarkers, and a laboratory career that focused on environmental health research, Michael was uniquely—perfectly—situated to study neurotoxins in ALS. He spent the next six years studying cyanobacteria, a blue-green algae, which has been linked to a higher incidence of ALS and other neurodegenerative diseases. With his eye-gaze computer, he analyzed data and emailed colleagues—up until his final days.

Pivot.

I had noticed this pattern with my ALS friends. Their ability to pivot. Just ordinary humans living ordinary lives until their ALS diagnosis. Then, despite their grief and sadness, they didn't lie down and give up. Not at all. Using their careers, skills, talents, or hobbies, they *pivoted* in extraordinary ways to make an impact with their remaining time. Like Chris Rosati, who "stole" the Krispy Kreme truck, then used the publicity and his marketing experience to launch his Inspire MEdia nonprofit.

I know this feeling, this pivot. It is the *why* behind all the marathons.

A recurring question continues to haunt me, though. Why do humans need a death sentence handed down in order to begin to *live*? To *pivot*? To have the audacity to pursue their highest calling?

After all, none of us are getting out of here alive.

Iowa and West Virginia:
Marathons #37 and #38
August 2021

The day before I was scheduled to leave for the Main to Main Marathon in northern Iowa (#37), I texted Shaw: "I have to pull out of the race." My planned travel companion had a COVID scare. David couldn't take off work; neither could Elizabeth.

The pressure was mounting with each race. I had been holding my breath waiting for something to go wrong. And now, with #37 on tap, it had.

"No way," Shaw said. "I will start driving your way at 5 A.M. We can make the flight."

And just like that, Shaw saved Iowa, and my fifty-state quest was still on track.

⌘

The next weekend, David and I met up with a few grad school friends, my parents, and my friend Leslie from Germany for the Moonlight on the Falls Marathon in West Virginia (#38).

West Virginia was my first-ever night marathon. Yes, night. As in middle of the night.

I learned much from the dark swamps of Florida. I brought a headlamp to West Virginia, along with fun green LED lights threaded through the spokes of my wheels. The fun green lights lasted; the headlamp did not.

The race started at 10 P.M. in the state park: four laps for a marathon. Once we got going, I realized how impossibly dark the race would be. No streetlights in the park meant I couldn't tell whether the road ahead was about to go up or down—and in West Virginia, the road is *always* going up or down.

I knew I was on a downhill only because the trike picked up speed. *Downhill, check. But how steep?* Steep enough and too dangerous to start flying like I normally would, was the answer. I had to be careful weaving around runners. Not everyone had lights.

When pedaling became difficult and lights bobbed past me, I was on an uphill. *Uphill, check. But how steep?* Each of the four loops was 668 feet, 2,672 feet total. More than twice as many as Montana. *I'm going to be out here all night!*

Then came an unexpected off-road section. *Oh. My. God.*

David and I had driven the course earlier but saw no indication of a gravel detour through the woods. I had no idea until I was *on it*. I couldn't see the path. I couldn't avoid the ruts. All I knew is that I was going *down*, because the trike was sliding down the gravel.

My heart rate spiked. I was downright terrified.

Going up, if you can believe it, was worse. The loose gravel shifted and slipped beneath the tires. I had no traction. In the dark, the normally helpful runner types couldn't see any sign of my struggle. My voice could not carry over the sound of crunching feet on the gravel.

All I could do was keep plowing ahead, praying for forward progress. *This has to end, just hang on.*

My friend Molly caught me near the top of the hill.

"You good?" she asked. Her headlamp illuminated my face, and she realized I wasn't good. But up ahead, I could see the headlights of a car, guiding runners. A car meant a road. *Pavement.* Sweet relief. I nodded to Molly. *But I cannot do that three more times!*

David rushed out to me as I finished the first loop.

"Molly said you needed help," he said. I was too shaken to talk for a minute. My parents ambled over. I would not admit defeat in front of them. Besides, I was in too deep now.

I explained the detour.

"Can you, um . . .?" I paused. I couldn't ask.

"You want me to go sit there, don't you," David said. It was not a question.

I looked up at him.

He sighed and said, "Yep."

⛬

The night and the loops wore on. The crowd thinned out as the half marathoners finished, which simultaneously offered relief and turned up the spooky factor. Just me and a few headlamps running through the West Virginia woods at night—*what could go wrong?*

Then my headlamp went out. *Well, shit. That's what.*

As if I needed more motivation to get this race over with. The quicker I finished, the less time David would have to sit out in the dark woods waiting for me.

"I keep seeing *eyes*," David said, as I skidded to his feet through the gravel for loop 2.

I tried to thank him, but he waved me off.

"Let's just get this done."

I knew David loved me. I asked a lot of him during the fifty marathons—that's for sure.

But West Virginia? Well, that was really the icing on the spooky cake. David sitting alone in the woods until 3 A.M. with *eyes* staring at him from the woods?

That is love.

July 2021

I still needed a Massachusetts race, so I turned my attention back to the Boston Marathon.

In 2019, the BAA became the first major marathon to rejig its divisions for athletes with physical and intellectual disabilities.[1] The BAA also created a new Adaptive Program, which allowed racers with a broad range of limitations to participate, including survivors who suffered injuries from the 2013 finish line bombing.

The new program was incredibly encouraging to me, because under these categories, athletes like me with impaired muscle power and hypertonia (increased muscle tone) could aspire to participate.

Even better? The BAA includes ALS (specifically) on the list of eligible impairments in order to race in one of the categories. *Wow!*

When I completed marathon #6 at the Publix Atlanta Marathon, I experienced some of the greatest moments of inclusion. I was so excited to see that Boston—one of the "majors" in the world marathon community—appeared to be making moves toward inclusion.

The BAA's changes recognized that runners with disabilities had the *same* reasons for racing as other runners: some wanted to be elite in their categories, some wanted to simply set goals and improve against their own performance, and others wanted to raise money for causes and charities.[2] They seemed to acknowledge that: each limitation or disability was different; each individual was different; and inclusion, therefore, would need to be handled on a case-by-case basis.

So, of course, I was excited. I was a unique case and I felt sure I could be included—bring on Boston!

But as I read the BAA's new adaptive rules, I wasn't sure what category applied to me. There were five categories for para athletes:

1. Wheelchair Division
2. Handcycle Program
3. Para Athletics Divisions—for competitive and world-class athletes
4. **Adaptive Program for Runners**
5. Duo Teams

I wasn't using a wheelchair or a handcycle, nor was I a world-class athlete (strike categories 1, 2, and 3). Nor was I looking to participate as a Duo Team, where I would be pushed in a racing chair (strike category 5).

Category 4, the new Adaptive Program for Runners, appeared to be where I fit. Plus, this category listed ALS as an "eligible impairment." Furthermore, the qualifying time for the Adaptive Program was 6:00:00—a time limit that I had never exceeded—not even once.*

There was one problem, though.

---

* Of the twenty-eight BQ marathons I'd finished, my slowest was Mississippi—the one where David ran four miles across town to fix my chain—and I still qualified with 4:59:39.

I wasn't running. I was pedaling a trike.

Still, I was encouraged about Boston as Marathon #50. I would show the BAA my story, qualifying times, and track record of safety. Since the ADA requires a "reasonable accommodation," I assumed the trike would be accepted. The only accommodations I needed were permission to participate in the only way I could—on my trike—and direction on when and where to line up. *Reasonable.*

Energized, I sent an email to the BAA in July 2021, excerpted below:

> *I am seeking to participate in the 2022 Boston Marathon through your Adaptive Program. . . . I was diagnosed with ALS 7 years ago at the age of 33. Since diagnosis, I have done* **41 full marathons in 36 states** *on my trike.*
>
> *Due to my impaired muscle strength, I do not have the coordination or upper body strength to use a push-rim wheelchair or handcycle . . . but my legs are still strong enough to self-propel the trike.*
>
> **My marathon times average between 3:30 and 4:30 . . .** *Typically, I start with the wheelchairs and push chairs so that the faster runners can see me to pass. I need no special assistance on the course, and safety is ALWAYS my priority. The largest marathon I have done is Philadelphia with 30,000 runners (close to Boston's numbers).*

While I received an encouraging initial response, ultimately I needed permission from the para athlete manager. I would not get an answer, however, until after the 2021 Boston Marathon, which had been rescheduled from April to October due to COVID.

Three months for an answer . . . and what if they said no?

Just in case Boston was a no, I would need a Massachusetts race (since I DNFed the one with the mini mountain). But no Massachusetts marathons take place over the winter for obvious reasons. And very few marathons are scheduled in the spring because of the Boston one in April.

Fortunately, I found one Massachusetts marathon that was eager to include me.

Massachusetts: Marathon #42
September 2021

The Martha's Vineyard Marathon (#42) would be my new MA insurance policy. I talked my matron of honor, Cathy, and her husband, Will, into coming with me. It would be Cathy's first half marathon.

Given the narrow trails in the first part of the marathon, the race director wanted me to start an hour early. No problem. I didn't mind that at all.

"If I can have everyone's attention," Michael, the barefoot, dread-headed emcee, announced to the crowd as I positioned at the start line. "This is Andrea Peet. Seven years ago, she was diagnosed with ALS. She has committed herself to doing a *marathon* in all fifty states. She has started her own foundation with all the funds going to ALS research. This is state number forty-two. So, I want everyone to come over, as close as you can, so we can give her some *love*."

The crowd erupted in cheers. *Well.* My name had been announced before an event, maybe even a reference to ALS or my goal, but never before had I been given such a *comprehensive* send-off. I was truly touched.

Massachusetts had become such an elusive medal—a goal within a goal—but this time, surely, victory was mine. But this darn state of Massachusetts? Well, I guess they relish a good fight. And Massachusetts wasn't ready to give up victory so easily.

At mile 2, my energy chews slipped out of my pocket. I had to circle back. At mile 6, a rain shower that I swear was only one cloud wide followed me around like a cartoon. I can't make this stuff up, but at least I saw a rainbow.

At mile 9, I crested a steep hill—big down, then big up. I took a deep breath, knowing I needed speed to reach the top. *Here we go. You can do this.*

Channeling another divebombing swallow, I flew down the hill, clocking 17 mph before the uphill slowed me down.

Pressing every ounce of strength into my quads, I made it almost to the top. *Almost.* And then my front wheels landed in a crack running the width of the paved trail. We're talking the Grand Canyon of cracks, enough to stop the trike—and me—cold. *Well, shit.*

At first I thought, *no problem. I know how to do this.*

I set my feet, deployed my trusty pedal-half-a-rotation technique, but the trike wouldn't budge. Too deep a crack, too little momentum. I tried again. Nothing. Again. Nothing.

It was ridiculous. All I'd been through, in forty-one marathons, only to be stymied by a crack in the pavement.

Maddening. Yet, the perfect microcosm of ALS—this crack. A fissure that someone without ALS wouldn't notice, yet impossible for someone with the disease to overcome.

When MJ and Brian realized my GPS point stopped moving, Brian came to find me with the camera. I had been stuck for ten minutes, swearing and attempting to clear the crack.

"What do you want me to do?" he asked, camera rolling. *Such a loaded question.*

After the mess I made of the New Orleans weekend, I was educated by MJ on a basic rule of documentary filmmaking.

Filmmakers are supposed to record the action, not *impact* it.

For example, if I am unable to get to a race start because handicap-accessible parking is blocked by construction, MJ and Brian are supposed to film this action—but not fix it by dropping me off at the start line.

Brian wasn't supposed to help me out of the crack.

At this point, I would have gladly accepted a push from another competitor, but the closest runner was forty minutes away.

"Well, at least you're here," I told him. "If I flip the trike, I flip." *Some extra drama for the documentary?* I preferred not to find out.

His question ("What do you want me to do?") provided the perfect motivation, though. *Not today, ALS.*

With one burst of power, I managed to get a half rotation out beyond the crack. That was all I needed. Brakes. Reset feet. One more burst of power for the back wheel to clear the crack. *Freedom!*

And that's just how you have to do it—life or marathons—sometimes. One foot in front of the other. When that's too much—stop, reset, and find the right impetus to keep fighting. Any forward progress is enough. One hard day, Hope will fight its way right into becoming *Belief.*

MJ believed it too, even without witnessing the crack incident. She met me at the finish line, camera in hand, her eyes shiny. "You are going to do this!" she said.

Oklahoma, New Jersey, and Delaware: Marathon #43, #44, and #46 October–November 2021

I cruised through the remaining fall races without further drama, collecting medals and memories.

The Oklahoma City Memorial Marathon (#43) honored victims of the Alfred P. Murrah Federal Building bombing in 1995. A wonderful tribute to a horrible tragedy.

Jillaine and I finished the Atlantic City Marathon (#44) together. She had been training all year to run the marathon in under four hours—"sub-4." We ticked off mile after mile with purpose. When her pace started to flag, I pulled just ahead of her so she could chase me. I wanted this goal for her more than any BQ time, and I urged her on in my head. *You got this, Jill. Just keep it up.* On the boardwalk in the final miles, we knew we'd done it. There is something magical about witnessing a friend achieve her dream, but it's even more fun to be along for the ride. We squeaked through the arch at 3:56, with our husbands cheering us in.

The last race of the year was in another boardwalk town: the Coastal Delaware Marathon (#46) in Rehoboth Beach. Ashley and I had completed the half together years before—right at the beginning of my ALS symptoms.

I marveled at how the town could change so little from that time, when I had changed so much.

Last time I was there, I was trying to accept that I was going to die. I had hoped for just one more race. I didn't understand it at the time, but Hope was pointing the way—from one race to another, like a series of stepping stones. One race, then another. And another. Hope revealed the path.

But I was the one who had taken the leap.

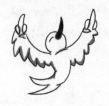

CHAPTER 34

THE BONUS
IN BOSTON

April 2022

The Martha's Vineyard Marathon checked off the state of Massachusetts for me. But I simply couldn't let go of the Boston Marathon.

I wanted to experience the full magic of this historic event. The whole city shuts down for that Monday in April—not for a national holiday—for a *marathon*. Bostonians are fiercely proud of their hometown race, even more so after the horrific Boston Marathon bombing. Boston Strong—I wanted to be part of it.

Spectators line both sides of the course from Hopkinton all the way to the Back Bay of Boston, screaming their heads off for complete strangers. I wanted to earn the medal and the coveted jacket with the Boston Marathon logo and three stripes down the arm. Heck, I wanted to do the infamous Heartbreak Hill, just to see for myself how bad it really was, betting secretly that I had scaled way tougher climbs in Montana and West Virginia.

After several more follow-up emails, I received a kindly worded denial in January 2022.

> *The BAA recognizes your effort, training, and desire to complete the Boston Marathon. Your story of overcoming ALS to finish more than 50 marathons is very special.*
>
> *While we understand your position as outlined in your email, we are unable to allow participation by way of a recumbent trike as that falls within a cycling realm. [Quoting the handcycle rules:] "No other gear, crank, or chain powered cycling equipment is permitted for use by athletes in the Boston Marathon including foot-powered recumbent bikes, tricycles, or bicycles."*

I had read and reread their quoted provision, but it still made no sense to me.

The handcycle (which is allowed) and trike (not allowed) both have three wheels and twenty-seven to thirty gears. I understood why the BAA needed to standardize handcycle equipment for that competitive category. Handcycles are typically ridden by a person who has lost one or both legs, or who is paralyzed below the waist. When I've started races next to handcycles, they are out of sight before I have cranked my legs around a couple of times. The BQ time for women handcyclists my age is 2:40:00, compared to my four-hour average.

Question: How is that possible? For someone to pedal faster with their hands than I can with my feet?

Answer: Because the typical handcyclist does *not* have functional disability in their upper body.

I'm not discounting the strength, training, or ability of a handcyclist. But I am pointing out that their disability is profoundly *different* from mine. They have lost ability in their legs (or have lost a limb entirely)—which necessitates the handcycle. But the neurological impact of my ALS affects the strength and coordination in my *entire* body.

The BAA allows for neurological impairments—listing ALS specifically as a qualifying impairment. They allow up to six hours to complete the course, which I have never needed. The only rule I don't meet is that I'm not *running*.

So, which is it, BAA? Am I too disabled, or not disabled enough? Because it's clearly not a safety issue. You allow faster mobility devices and slower runners. You are never going to write a rule to address all physical manifestations of all disabilities.

What is wrong with a case-by-case review?

And, even better, you have the power to *invite* anyone to participate that you wish. In fact, you have approximately six thousand of those spots with your charity program and special passes for sponsors, vendors, and the like.

You can *invite* individuals who have overcome extraordinary circumstances and have a proven safety track record. You can invite athletes who are racing at their highest level of *ability*—thereby providing Hope to others that they too can aspire to participate in the Boston Marathon.

The sheer action of consideration, individual analysis, and then *invites* would be a glowing beacon in the right direct toward inclusion. Although it doesn't nearly cover comprehensive inclusion, it would be a start. History shows we have to start somewhere—and from the top.

Eyes on you, Boston.

⁂

Oh, how I tried to let it go. *You don't need Boston anymore,* I told myself. *Focus on the gratitude for all the marathons that have let you in. You don't need to fight this battle. Rules are rules. Stupid rules, but rules.*

Rules are rules. I'd always been a rule follower. A goody-goody.

The BAA's damn rule *grated* on me, though.

I mean, women weren't allowed to participate in Boston until 1972. Rules are rules.

And there we were, in 2022, with the BAA loudly celebrating the fiftieth anniversary of women officially being allowed to run the Boston Marathon. *Women, but not me.*

"I don't think the BAA understands just how hard it is for you, with ALS, to even *show up* to a race," my friend Jess said.

The BAA had the right to decide who could run their marathon, but they didn't own the streets of Massachusetts.

They could keep me out of the Boston Marathon, but if I wanted to race the course, no one could stop me.

And that's just what I did. The day before the actual event.

⁂

By the time our crew arrived in Boston two days before the actual race, the Back Bay was already an anthill of activity and anticipation—runners, spectators, and vendors crawling all over each other to take care of last-minute purchases, meet up with friends, and attend panel discussions with celebrity runners. The Boston Strong motto was out in full force—everyone had earned their spot.

Except me.

I felt like an imposter even being in the frenzy of the pre-race days. *What the hell was I thinking?*

There was a screening of short documentaries and a panel discussion put on by the Brooks running company. The documentary series, titled "Who Is a Runner," featured the Chinatown Runners group formed during the pandemic, a queer runner, a woman running to call attention to missing and murdered Indigenous women, and the Prolyfyck Run Crew, a Black-led running group in Charlottesville, Virginia.

Anna Katherine Clemmons, a freelance journalist writing a story about me for the *New York Times*, met us at the panel. She had written pieces about Prolyfyck and wanted to introduce us to Will Jones III.

In the wake of the white supremacist rally in Charlottesville, Will began organizing community runs through predominately Black neighborhoods. Everyone was welcome, and the group sometimes had more than sixty runners of all racial, ethnic, and running backgrounds cheering each other along.

"It's important that you are able to look out in the world and *see yourself* to give you some courage," Will says in the documentary.

Although our inclusion issues were totally different, I nodded along. That's what I wanted people to see, too.

An ALS diagnosis was essentially being told there was no Hope for your future. No cure, no treatment, no chance of recovery. That hopelessness is killer, even faster than the ALS itself. But what if seeing me do fifty marathons—even a single marathon, and especially the Boston Marathon—could be enough to give someone with ALS a little bit of Hope? A permission, if you will, to ask of themselves: "If she can do it, then why not me?" Or perhaps, "What can I still push my body to do?"

"We decide to push through the fear. That's what makes us brave," Will says.

I knew what I had to do. Sitting in the audience, I hit "publish" on the social media post I had been carrying around all day.

It read, "I'm just not as willing to accept 'no' anymore."

⊷≫∘

The next day, the day before the *real* Boston Marathon, the filmmakers met us at 5 A.M. for the ride to Hopkinton. With no sidewalks for the first few miles of the course, we needed to be out early, before traffic picked up.

Even so, I delayed the start by fifteen minutes while David wrote on our car's back window: MY OWN BOSTON MARATHON.

David and I had negotiated for a month about how this would work. "I'll just ride with a couple of bike escorts," I said, wanting to do my own race.

"There's no way I'm not driving behind you," he said.

Since the filmmakers also needed to be close, I agreed.

"But no flashers," I said.

"Flashers," he said, firmly.

When I sent out an email asking for a couple of bike escorts, our entourage grew to four bikes and two cars (with flashers). Two of the cyclists were scientists from ALS TDI, one of whom woke up at 2:30 A.M. to bike out to Hopkinton.

I took a deep breath.

"Go?" I said, having never started myself in a race before.

My entourage and I rolled over the yellow-and-blue start line painted across the road for the real Boston Marathon start the next day.

As always, the rhythm of the marathon calmed my nerves. My fears about traffic, logistics, and royally pissing off the BAA melted away through my quads and my feet as I pedaled. Aside from the occasional passing car, the world was quiet as dawn broke.

No one cared that we were out there.

But I care. And that was enough.

As we passed metal barriers stacked up like pancakes for the race, I tried to picture the crowds of spectators I'd seen on TV. I looked for the spray-painted mile markers and pretended I was surrounded by thousands of thudding feet. I waved at cars when we got a few honks of encouragement.

Up ahead, I heard a cowbell and could see a figure jumping up and down. My heart skipped a beat—Carol Hamilton, the VP of development for ALS TDI.

Now, I adore Carol. As a fundraiser myself, I have studied her moves and constantly marvel at how she can be so poised, sincere, and irreverent, all at once, in a way that makes donors practically throw their money at her. She cares passionately about curing ALS. When an aquarium tried to lure her away with a lucrative job offer, she said, matter-of-factly: "My friends are dying and you want me to care about *fish*?"

"Goooo, Andrea! See you at the finish line!" she cried. I almost cried.

The first fifteen miles of the Boston Marathon are a net downhill with a few rollers. Even with those modest hills, the BAA's contention that the trike was too far into the "cycling realm" became laughable. I pushed every available leg muscle to its limit, trying not to embarrass myself, as my escorts on their two-wheeled road bikes looped lazy circles around me. Up the hill, down the hill, back and forth, calling out encouragements as they passed. I tried to respond but was huffing and puffing too hard. This was no joke.

So, I smiled.

Every day I get to do this is a good day, I repeated to myself. Followed shortly by, *Cycling realm, my ass.*

At Heartbreak Hill,* my entourage reshuffled. The filmmakers positioned themselves for the finish, and David joined me for what would amount to a slow walk up a long hill. Anna Katherine Clemmons from the *New York Times* showed up, too.

With a name like Heartbreak, I wasn't sure how steep of a hill I was in for. I wanted David with me in case I got in trouble.

I was relieved. It was steep, but doable. No Martha's Vineyard–sized cracks in the pavement either.

I narrowed my eyes and fixed them on a mailbox a few yards away. I reeled it in. Slow, steady, patient. One foot in front of the other.

Then the next mailbox. No need to freak out. *I can do this.*

---

* The famed Heartbreak Hill gets its name from the 1936 race at the point when Johnny Kelley overtook Ellison "Tarzan" Brown to win the marathon. It's half-mile climb toward Mile 21, the fourth in a series of uphills, and the last major hill before the finish. In other words, heartbreaking to exhausted runners.

That's all this journey is. That's all any journey is. One race at a time, one hill at a time, one foot at a time.

I breathed hard, grateful I still could. I was still an athlete—stronger than ALS. I was more than proud. I was confident.

Cresting the top of Heartbreak, the iconic landmarks of Boston came into view—the Prudential Tower and Fenway *Pahk*. Just as millions of Boston Marathoners before me, I felt my spirit and pace lift.

Poor David. He had poked along slowly with me as I churned my legs, ignoring him and staring down mailboxes. But at the top, I just said, "See ya!" I felt my wheels gathering speed before I began hurtling down the hill. *Totally obnoxious.*

"Get it! I love you!" he yelled to my back as I picked up speed. That is our marriage. He will worry, but he will never hold me back.

A few minutes later, I heard "Keep it up, Andrea!" from someone on the sidewalk wearing a blue-and-yellow Boston Marathon finisher jacket. *Who is that?* The face looked familiar but totally out of context. I waved and smiled.

I didn't know it at the time, but Carol had used her charming I'm-going-to-get-you-to-do-whatever-I-want sweet talk on the Boston police officers around the finish line. By the time she finished telling my story, the officers had agreed to clear the way for me to cross the finish line of My Own Boston Marathon.

As we turned the corner onto Boylston Street, the police hustled the runner-tourists taking selfies at the finish line out of our way.

Suddenly, our entourage doubled in size. No, tripled. My eyes couldn't take it all in at once. David—the guy is fast—reappeared by my side. Jess, who would be running the marathon the next day, showed up in her Team Drea knitted cap, along with her friends, bike escorts, filmmakers, friends I had expected to see and friends I hadn't, total strangers, Anna Katherine, and a pack of runners I recognized from the documentary film panel the day before—*oh my gosh, Prolyfyck!*

Will Jones III started a chant: "Tell it to go!" and the others finished, "The body will go!"

"Tell it to go! The body will go!"

Soon all the runner-tourists on Boylston Street started clapping for us. Because that's what runners do. *Boston Strong.*

"Tell it to go! The body will go!" And in that moment, I believed them and bought into the magic.

ALS is such a mindfuck. ALS bodies, for the most part, won't go, even as hard as you will them to. The brain-nerve-muscle connection is gone. You can't create something from nothing.

But for me, in that moment, I had something. My body could still go.

All I had was that moment. And that was enough. And no one could take it away.

The noise was absolutely deafening as I crossed the finish line. My body was consumed with joy. Absolutely overwhelmed.

I didn't bother trying to speak. With fist bumps, hugs, and a hand over my heart, I tried to convey my gratitude to the Prolyfyck runners and my friends around me.

Out of the corner of my eye, I saw a blue-and-yellow Boston finisher jacket, the person who had cheered me on from the sidewalk. *Now* I recognized who it was. And I could scarcely believe it.

Ryan Auster.

A rower in my boat.

From college.

Whom I hadn't seen in twenty years.

I waved him over, coupled with a wide-eyed shake of my head and shrug. The universal what-the-hell-are-you-doing-here gesture.

"I know you aren't able to run tomorrow," he said, pulling something out of his pocket. A blue-and-yellow ribbon unfurled.

A Boston Marathon medal. Everyone gasped.

"You just did the Boston Marathon, and you deserve a medal," Ryan said, placing it around my neck while my friends cheered.

The tears came, just as they still do every time I think of his kindness. It would have been enough just to see him, that he came to see me. But the medal? It was too much. I couldn't speak.

"It doesn't say the right year," he said, and we all laughed.

When I regained my composure, he crouched down to my level so we could talk.

"I saw your post," he said. "I live forty-five minutes away. I had to come."

I shook my head, trying to wrap my mind around all that had happened. How does such beautiful kindness exist in a world of such brutality, or even distracted indifference?

The wholeness of that moment was complete. Everyone felt the power, but no one could feel the best of humanity reverberating from all sides quite like I could.

Jon Blais knew. I knew. *Again*.

And that's how the marathon I wasn't allowed to do became one of my favorite memories of all time.

CHAPTER 35

AN ATTEMPT AT THE IMPOSSIBLE

Nevada: Marathon #47
January 2022

My friend Jess and I were on edge.

Our early flight arrival into Vegas *plus* a new COVID variant *plus* the trike damaged by the airlines *again*—well, it hadn't been a stress-free morning.

Our anxiety levels dropped as we drove out of Las Vegas. Red rock boulders replaced the strip malls. The air felt somewhat lighter, the sky bluer.

Still, we were *edgy*.

Which might explain our audible gasps of wonder as Lake Mead appeared on the horizon: a massive lake—oddly out of place in the middle of the desert—ringed by burnt-red mountains with vast blue sky above. I did a double take to make sure it wasn't a mirage.

Lake Mead Marathon (#47) took place on the trail skirting the lake, just a short drive from the Hoover Dam. Jess had planned to run the half marathon but sprained her ankle the week before the race. Thankfully, she came on the trip to help me with, well, everything outside of the marathon.

My last drops of anxiety evaporated as I started pedaling. *Logistics: done. Trike: fixed. Speaking: not necessary. Worries: gone.* I realized Lake Mead was the last race where I'd be out in the wild, all alone. The last three races—Oakland, Brooklyn, even Alaska—would be surrounded by crowds, filmmakers, celebrations—all amazing, but would demand a lot from me. Nevada would be my own personal celebration, I decided. *Party of one. Let four hours of freedom begin!*

The desert landscape fascinated me, foreign to my life as an East Coaster and even unique to my fifty-state journey. I'd seen cacti in Arizona. I'd seen dry land in Wyoming. I'd seen red rocks in New Mexico. But this area was parched dry, almost completely devoid of vegetation. The few scorched-looking scrub bushes didn't look like vegetation at all.

Then I spotted a small, purple wildflower growing in a gutter at the bottom of a hill.

The purple flower wasn't showy, just out of place. I only caught a glimpse before I rolled past. But the image stuck in my mind and gave me questions to ponder for miles. *How could it grow there? Randomly? Out of a seam in the concrete?*

But what a perfect spot it was.

The bottom of the hill was where any water—no matter how little existed—collected. The water must have brought enough soil and sediment for a seed to root. The seed certainly didn't choose that location. Who would?

But in those bottom-of-the-gutter conditions, a seed sprouted. Through all the harsh desert conditions, the seedling hung on, and fought for its life.

Against all odds, it found a way to bloom.

The best part? That flower would spread seeds, carrying incrementally better wisdom of how to survive the unforgiving climate. The seeds just needed a chance to do it for themselves.

California: Marathon #48
March 2022

Almost three years to the day after COVID derailed our original plan, we made it to California. *Thirty marathons later.*

My new friend Peggy met us at the Oakland Marathon (#48) for her first race since being diagnosed with ALS.

Peggy had been a pre-elite gymnast, then a collegiate diver. As an adult, she had run the Chicago Marathon twenty years in a row for charity. The day Peggy received the crushing diagnosis, she went home and did an internet search. Having heard there was a greater incidence of the disease among endurance athletes, Peggy typed in a search for "marathon running" and "ALS."

But instead of scientific journal articles, my story popped up.

"When I read your story, I thought to myself, 'Well, I'm getting a Catrike too!'" she said.

That bright line stretching from Jon Blais to me . . . now extended to Peggy.

"It's so fun to be part of a race again!" Peggy said, as we pedaled the first 10K together.

After the finish, I saw a woman sitting on a rollator—a walker with four wheels, a seat, and brakes. Maybe because we were at eye level, or maybe because I'm not used to seeing women my age using a walker, I stared a half second too long. Consequently, we locked eyes, then smiled, then waved, then struck up a conversation.

Mary had a different neurological disease, one I'd only heard about because it was mentioned as a possibility for me early on. She knew all about ALS, though. Her grandmother—the one she was named after—had died from ALS.

She asked me a bunch of questions about my trike.

The next day Mary messaged me on social media and told me she was thinking about getting a trike. She did, and in her first half marathon, she raised $1,000 for Team Drea in honor of her grandmother.

❦

A couple years earlier, Mom and I had toured the Catrike factory in Orlando while in town for an ALS conference.

The assembly line area was almost a spiritual experience for me. Like walking through a trike nursery. Being surrounded by half-built trikes and containers of bolts, springs, levers, and other parts moved me in the best way.

You're going to change someone's life. And you are. And you too, I telegraphed silently to each of the little baby trikes.

Not going to lie, I teared up.

Thinking about Mary and Peggy, I realized I was like that little flower in Nevada. Stranded in the arid land of ALS, against all odds, I had bloomed in an adorable green trike. ALS is still brutal, still kills most people far too quickly. But. *I cannot be the only one out there like me.* The wisdom I've acquired about staying strong through exercise can help others. It already has. Those baby trike seeds are starting to spread, carried along by the wind and the waters of Hope.

New York: Marathon #49
April 2022

For the film, it was important to introduce someone with advanced ALS.

I had assumed that my own progression during filming would show the cruelty of the disease. But even during the years of filming, the changes to my voice and gait were subtle from a cinematic standpoint—which, of course, I was grateful for.

But we needed to be clear about what ALS does to the human body.

ALS is *not* all marathons and rainbows.

Remember that the average life expectancy is only two to five years from diagnosis—with a broad spectrum of quality of life in those two to five years. Yes, *thankfully*, I was progressing slowly. Yes, *thankfully*, my mission of Hope was rolling along.

But I am an extreme outlier.

ALS is heartless. ALS is cruel. ALS is inhumane. Everyone needs to understand the horrific nature of ALS, no matter how hard it might be to see (or read).

An awkward request, though—asking someone to be in your film because they are suffering more visibly than you are. *Ugh.* "Hey, can we come stick cameras in your face because you're so much more worse off than I am? Oh, and I'm finishing marathons too. That's what the film is about." *Double ugh.*

I felt the typical-to-Andrea wave of guilt wash over me—but pushed it away. I reminded myself that guilt was a waste of time. Then I had a lightbulb moment.

I knew exactly who to ask.

In our documentary titled "Go On, Be *Brave*," I knew my audience must meet the *bravest* person I knew: Mayuri Saxena. Who just happened to live near the Brooklyn Marathon (#49).

Mayuri had typed her memoir with her eyes via computer. Her book, *The Pursuit of Happiness: From Heels to Wheels*, outlined her story as a first-generation American born to Indian parents. Her carefree years growing up in the melting pot of New York City came to an abrupt halt following September 11, 2001. Even with two master's degrees and a security clearance, Mayuri encountered thinly veiled prejudice in the wake of 9/11. She was fired from her federal job. Her young marriage fell apart. Then, her leg began twitching—leading to her ALS diagnosis. All before she turned thirty-three.

As adventurous as I am, I'm a damn wallflower next to Mayuri.

A quick rundown of things I would never attempt, but Mayuri has successfully accomplished: commuting regularly to work via wheelchair on the NYC subway, embarking on a *solo* international trip in a wheelchair to five countries (some not exactly known for accessibility—like India and Egypt), and posting glamorous photos from professional yet bedridden photo shoots.

So, I asked Mayuri to be the one to show the world how ALS typically affects the human body. Of course, in her fabulous Mayuri style, she agreed. Mayuri welcomed David, the filmmakers, and me into her home for the interview.

On her social media and featured in the documentary are photos of Mayuri, pre-ALS and early on in her progression, as she traveled around the world. She was stunning—perfect makeup, gorgeous saris.

But that day in her home, I witnessed—once again—all that ALS had taken away. What living with a trach truly entailed. She hadn't left her bed in three years due to COVID fears—except for trach changes, which required an ambulance ride to the hospital.

Every few minutes, she said (through her eye-gaze computer): "Suction."

On that command, a home health aide thrust a tube in her mouth and a loud machine sucked out excess saliva. Without constant monitoring, Mayuri would choke. I watched and thought, *I can't imagine this level of vulnerability.* I knew from Mayuri's social media that this vulnerability was a constant source of stress for her too. Some aides were more attentive than others. She has had several close calls. This help wasn't cheap either. Every few months, her brother appealed on social media for financial assistance, for the money to simply keep Mayuri alive.

Yet, I also witnessed what ALS hadn't taken. From her hospital bed in the living room, Mayuri has also launched her most impactful campaigns to date. Without the ability to talk, eat, breathe on her own, or move anything except her eyes, Mayuri has hosted sock drives for the homeless, organized elaborate birthday parties, and is taking college-level physics classes from Arizona State University. She has become more deeply focused on her meditation practice. As David and I sat talking to her, she secretly ordered brightly colored rainbow bagels so I could carb-load before the race.

In 2020 and 2021, Mayuri lobbied Congress to pass the ACT for ALS: the most expansive funding and programmatic bill to date to support ALS and other rare neurological diseases.

Mayuri posted:

> ALS is a disease that will challenge your ego, and ultimately wins unless you take your own life. I slowly started to accept if I was going to survive another day, that I would have to allow others to bathe me, clean me, and even feed me. Then the biggest blow came when I had my tracheostomy. I officially lost my voice, and lost a bit of myself during the process. . . .
>
> But my purpose became more clear as I stopped feeling sorry for myself. . . .
>
> I knew I could give back to my community, and started advocating with just my eyes. . . . Finally, I accepted what I knew all along—that I am a warrior at heart, and this is my journey.

Mayuri was on my mind all the next day as I tackled the Brooklyn Marathon. I drew strength from her spirit. Not pity. Strength. *If Mayuri is brave enough to live a meaningful life from bed and accomplish all she has with just her eyes, you can damn sure power up this hill.*

Being brave means using our abilities—whatever they may be—to live our fullest lives possible, to live past our fear.

Alaska: Marathon #50
May 2022

Dr. Bedlack told the filmmakers in an interview that my goal for fifty marathons was "an attempt at the impossible."

Remember, he's the Doctor of Hope. He's been one of my biggest cheerleaders since the first day I met him. So, he certainly never expressed any doubts to *me*.

I heard his words in an interview with the filmmakers—almost three years later. When I *personally* told Dr. Bedlack about my goal, he said to me: "If you get to fifty marathons, I will be there at the finish line in Boston."

Even though it wasn't Boston, Dr. Bedlack remained true to his word. The final trip to the final marathon on Prince of Wales Island required three planes, two ferries, and an hour's drive to a remote island in southeastern Alaska. Dr. Bedlack joined a group of forty-seven others: family members, Team Drea friends, and an expanded film crew.*

Basically, it felt like a wedding or the Team Drea party—except this time I was determined not to freak out. David and I leaned heavily on our Team Drea Alaska committee to plan this last, most complicated, trip.

It was the *finale* to the *impossible*, after all.

The committee tackled everything, from transportation to tours for hiking, fishing, and whale-watching to race day volunteer duties. They nailed details that never occurred to me—like walkie-talkies for the lack of cell service—and planned a Beer Mile (one beer every quarter mile). They also managed to pull off so many special, personal touches I'd envisioned—like a rock-painting station so we could add to the local tradition of leaving painted rocks on trails for others to find.

Shaw used her Team Drea superpowers from home. She hosted the video livestream for the finish line and organized our massive $50,000 fundraising campaign: the ALS 50for50 Challenge in the fifty days leading up to Alaska.

The 50for50 Challenge posed the question: "What's your brave?"

---

* In attendance: David, my parents, Dr. Dave, Elizabeth, Jillaine and Jodi, Cathy and Will and their son (our godson) Luke, Molly and other grad school friends with me for that crazy night race in West Virginia, my Pilates instructor Mischa, Peggy and her trike, Carol from ALS TDI, and an assortment of friends from high school, college, and every other corner of my life.

We asked people to "be brave *your* own way" by selecting a physical or personal goal around the number fifty and donating at least fifty dollars for ALS research. Some of our suggestions: walk fifty miles, meditate for fifty days, do fifty random acts of kindness. More than two hundred people registered and took on more creative challenges than I ever anticipated.

Elizabeth—a notoriously picky eater—posted hilarious videos of attempting fifty new foods (nothing exotic—we are talking strawberries, grapes, and tomato soup). She donated fifty dollars for every food she didn't finish. Jess created swallow bird art each day for fifty days. My niece drew fifty very smart cats curing ALS.

Team Drea, in appreciation for completing the challenge, mailed participants the most Drea thing I could conjure: a race medal with a mirror as the center. *What's your brave? All you have to do is look in the mirror.* I'm super cheesy like that.

❦

Before we left, MJ and Brian filmed our packing process for Alaska.

This "process" consisted of David and me cramming entirely too many things into suitcases. From swag to rock-painting supplies, we had it all—including special finale marathon T-shirts. The front of the shirt read, simply, BRAVE. But the *V* was a ponytailed figure in a trike, throwing her arms up the way I always do when I cross the finish line. *V for victory.*

"Can you put into words what Alaska means to you?" MJ asked as we packed, camera rolling.

I couldn't. I stumbled over my words.

She tried another angle. "What are you most excited about?"

I lit up. That was easy. "For my friends to meet each other!"

Not everyone on Team Drea knew each other in person, and I was thrilled for them to meet. But also, I was connecting my community with another community that had been waiting to welcome us for over two years. I alone knew how amazing and special each person was—on Team Drea and on POW.*

---

* Yes, Prince of Wales uses the acronym "POW". Yes, I know, I thought "prisoner of war" too the first dozen times I read it. Welcome to Alaska! They do what they want—in the best ways.

When the two worlds collided in one place? Would we break the matrix? Would a new portal to awesomeness open up?

"What are you most worried about?" MJ asked.

Another easy one.

"My voice," I said.

Lately, I had to concentrate more than ever to articulate my words, to press my mouth muscles into the right shapes to form the sounds. My sluggish tongue rarely felt like cooperating. My speech was worse when I was tired. I couldn't imagine my voice after six days straight of gabbing with friends, speaking to five school groups, and serving as the guest speaker for the pre-race dinner.

(At least that would all happen before I had to—you know—do a marathon.) *Yikes.*

To make matters worse, I had developed a mental block.

I already knew I talked slowly. I knew my speech was slurred. People with ALS are well aware of their failing bodies. There's nothing wrong with our minds. We just find ourselves trapped in bodies that refuse to cooperate.

So, because I *knew* I was having speech issues, my internal anxiety decided to compound the issue. Like when you're wearing high heels or when you're walking across the stage at graduation and you whisper to yourself, "Don't trip, don't trip, don't trip," and then *SPLAT*. Same thing.

When I became nervous or anxious, my speech was even worse. I found myself hung up on long or hard-to-pronounce words—especially when giving presentations or talking to reporters. Like a stutter, except I froze.

All I could do was follow my own advice. Repeat to myself what I had been telling Team Drea for almost eight years. Repeat to myself my call to action for the 50for50 Challengers.

Go on, be brave.

Be scared and go for it anyway.

⌒⌒⌒

"How do you know Andrea?"

This question was the icebreaker upon everyone's arrival in Prince of Wales. It worked so well that soon my Team Drea and POW friends were hiking and painting rocks together, singing and carrying on over bottles of wine. A very particular kind of magical fairy dust had been sprinkled over our group. Everyone got along, everyone pitched in, no one complained.

The rustic, beautiful scenery in the tiny Alaskan town of Klawock oozed adventure and wilderness and jaw-dropping scenery for the week we were there leading up to Memorial Day.

The big picture window at our home base, the Fireweed Lodge, framed our view of the water, the dock, and the Fireweed's fishing boats. Across the sound, an evergreen forest flanked the base of a snow-covered mountain. Once, we watched a fat black bear lumber out at low tide to do some fishing. Overhead, bald eagles swooped and yelled at each other. These majestic, protected symbols of freedom appeared as frequently as breakfast. Everything felt glorious, yet common; magical, but just as it should be.

The Fireweed served up mouthwatering fresh seafood followed by an endless dessert bar. In between her duties as manager, Chace pulled out her guitar and played a few songs; her six-year-old son Jax belted out the words to "Wagon Wheel."

This trip, I had built downtime into my schedule. I didn't need to relearn any lessons about overscheduling. So, sometimes during the day, I'd curl up on the oversized leather couch overlooking the water. I breathed. I rested. I dreamed. I talked to whoever wandered in to make themselves a sandwich.

My school group appearances began on a Wednesday in the nearby town of Craig. I corralled David into tag-teaming the presentations with me, just in case my voice became an issue. We brought temporary tattoos that said "Go On, Be Brave" with eight swallows for all the students, divided up into little plastic baggies for the teachers to distribute.

Craig Elementary's baggie had twenty-one tattoos for the first-grade class; Klawock's upper school (middle and high school combined) baggie had forty tattoos. These schools were tiny compared to my high school of two thousand students. I worried we wouldn't be able to connect with them. *What do I know about talking to kids?*

We told my story through photos in the gym and auditorium of the respective schools. David explained that ALS was like a telephone from your brain calling your muscles to tell them what to do. I thought it was the perfect analogy. Only later I realized that the phones these kids were familiar with, even in a small town in Alaska, likely had no cords attached.

Our last picture slide was a photo of my tattooed arm.

"I want to leave you with a message of hope," I said. "No matter what goes wrong or how hard it seems, there is always hope. You just need to go on and be brave."

The kids were respectful and asked great questions. Still, it was hard to know whether the message landed. My voice had held up, so that was as good as it could be, I guessed.

⤜⥈⤛

The race weekend, in POW style, added special touches, too.

The pre-race spaghetti dinner was a party. Swallows adorned the windows of Craig High School where we gathered. Elementary students performed a Native people's song; some classes had worked together on a poster, coloring a halibut for each racer. A flash mob appeared and started the electric slide. Of course, many Team Drea members jumped in.

David and I had planned to tag-team an adult version of our school presentation for the conclusion of the dinner, but just before we approached the podium, I turned to him.

"I got this. I'm just going to talk, okay?" I whispered. His eyes widened, then he nodded.

(He says this is one of his favorite Alaska memories.)

I spoke from the heart about bravery, and community, and how much it meant to have so many friends with us to celebrate this milestone—especially on the eighth anniversary of my diagnosis. Hard to believe that eight years ago, I fell and smacked my lip on the carpet before hearing the words *probable ALS* for the first time.

When Dr. Bedlack and Carol Hamilton from ALS TDI finished their remarks, David and I returned to the podium.

We presented each of them with donations from the 50for50 Challenge—for $50,000 apiece. Their mouths dropped open in surprise.

(This is one of *my* favorite Alaska memories.)

In the fifty days leading up to the marathon, our campaign had doubled its goal and raised $100,000 for ALS research.

And *that* is the power of community coming together.

⤜⥈⤛

Seeing Peggy in her trike at the start line brought me a little rush of joy. And fear.

Her ALS had advanced measurably since Oakland—*had that really been only two months ago?* Her local bike shop had moved all the trike shifting to the left side; her right hand no longer had strength to push or pull a lever. The Oakland 10K had been much flatter than the half marathon hills of Prince of Wales. So, I worried.

At least she gets to turn around before the madness really starts. Having driven the out-and-back course with David and the filmmakers, I knew the marathon course was tough. I knew it might be the hardest one of all, aside from West Virginia. *At least it will be daylight. And no way will I DNF my fiftieth marathon.*

The POW Marathon began the countdown to start Peggy and me. I refused to let in any thoughts about this being my "last race." (I thought about that Ramblin' Rose triathlon—and look what had happened!)

At the same time, I couldn't deny that my knees and hips and toes had been beat up with the pace of my sprint to Alaska. Was that ALS progression or athletic wear and tear? Both, I suspected.

Instead, I focused on the gratitude of my communities coming together, the money we had raised for ALS research, and the incredible, *insane* journey leading up to that moment.

Today, you can still do this.

✺

The first half of the race was filled with welcome distractions. Even with low clouds in the sky, I created countless Alaskan postcards in my mind. The snowy mountain ranges, the rugged trees jutting out of the water's edge. *So quintessentially Alaskan*, I thought, even with no other reference points for comparison. *Such an Oregon problem to have. So Florida. Just like Massachusetts. This has been an adventure like no other.*

The roads were open to traffic, so I found myself waving at all the honking horns. Supportive residents, vans filled with Team Drea, kids' relay vans. *Beep beep beep!* Cheering and clapping.

Some of my waving opportunities and appreciated distractions:

- The schools had organized fifteen-person relay teams made up of kindergarteners through sixth graders. The kid runner charged full speed—alone—on the side of the highway for more than a mile, while the van leapfrogged up to the next exchange point. Then all the kids piled out of the van to receive the runner, cheering their little hearts out. *Absolutely adorable.* I felt a little burst of pride. *Like Mom probably feels watching me achieve my dreams.* And my breath caught. I appreciated her now more than ever.
- Team Drea racers running the half marathon, heading back for the finish.
- Our eight-person relay team, identifiable by the capes they'd brought for the occasion.
- The twenty-six signs posted along the route at every mile marker. Each sign had a photo and short bio to honor a Team Drea loved one lost too soon to ALS, or my friends with ALS and those who had inspired me (Jon Blais was mile 1; I was mile 26).

Around mile 9, David and the filmmakers began to walk with me. The elevation had really picked up. I had encountered steeper slopes in Austin and in Montana, but the Alaskan hills seemed to go on for an eternity.

I flew on the downhills, happy for the short respite. But also with the sinking realization that any hill I coasted down would be another climb on the way back.

I was losing time off the 4:30 finish time I'd predicted to Shaw, who was operating the livestream for the folks back home. I had a short pang of guilt, then promptly shook it off. I was working as hard as I could. *Guilt is a wasted emotion.*

"Knees not happy," I said to David, breathing hard. The back of my left knee had been swollen for weeks, even with massages from Mischa to disperse the fluid buildup and bring healing to the area. As much strength as we'd built in Pilates, it was no match for these Alaska hills—or, apparently, ALS.

"Tell it to go! The body will go!"

I smiled, mimicking Prolyfyck's chant from Boston. That memory made me smile big enough to keep digging—I had to find joy in the struggle. *My fiftieth marathon. The hardest yet. Would I really want it any other way?*

"I need some real food at the next aid station," I wheezed at David a few minutes later. "Carbs."

I was running on empty. MJ, walking next to us and filming, said later that it was at this point she knew I was really struggling.

As we trudged up the worst of the hills, a two-mile slog that just wouldn't let up, we saw people pile out of a van up ahead.

All people unmistakably wearing BRAVE shirts. *MY people!*

And they were *exactly* who I needed to see right then: Jenny, Deb, and Lori—all ALS widows. They had been out on the course to take photos with Team Drea signs honoring their late husbands. Alongside them was Carol from ALS TDI and Colette. Colette had previously worked at ALS TDI but left the organization when her best friend—the brilliant Sarah Coglianese—passed away from ALS.

"This disease, it's so fucking brutal," Colette said when she was interviewed for the film. I love her delightful Irish accent, along with her equally delightful Irish propensity to swear every other sentence. "I'm not strong enough to keep doing what the people at ALS TDI do every day." (She says that, but she adds to the swallow tattoo collection on her arm every year when I do. And she immediately said yes to coming to Alaska. She is that kind of friend.)

"Colette!" David yelled ahead to her. "Get her up this hill with your Tri-State Trek routine!"

One year at ALS TDI's bike ride, I impulsively decided to attempt the legendary John Street hill, a 13-percent-grade monster that only some riders can successfully summit—the rest end up walking their bikes to the top.

Like a drill sergeant, Colette had gotten down in my face, yelling and swearing her encouragement while I slowly cranked forward at a snail's pace. She made damn sure I wouldn't quit, and I loved her for it.

She was up to the job now, too.

She got in position to walk beside me.

"C'mon, you got this. Stop letting down, go," Colette said, next to my ear. Then she bellowed, "ONE! TWO! THREE!" I started laughing and fought just that much harder. *Talk about full circle,* I thought. *She is coxswaining me!*

"Do you see it?" she pointed to the top of the hill.

I nodded my helmet vigorously, laughing. "DO YOU SEE IT? You're fucking invincible is what you are. COME ON!"

The other women chimed in, singing the Rocky theme song loudly.

A team effort, as it had been all along. ALS had taken so much from us all—and yet, it brought us together. To this island. To this hill. To this memory none of us will ever forget.

⊰⊱

An hour later, cruising down the last hill, I passed the mile 26 sign with my photo. *How many times had I imagined this moment?*

"Do you think you'll cry at the finish?" David had asked me.

"Nah," I had said. "You know me. I won't be able to stop smiling."

Grinning from ear to ear, I made the last turn and saw the finish arch in front of Craig High School. As I made my way up the last hill of all fifty states (because of course there was a hill), the cheering began.

Racers, the POW community, and Team Drea lined the finish chute. I fist-bumped Peggy, who had finished her half marathon. *Yes! Go, Peggy!*

My teammates, my dear friends, my parents—each held out one of the other forty-nine race medals that had gotten me to this point. *Forty-nine (well, plus My Own Boston) marathons. Fifty-one marathons. Here I am.*

Such pandemonium. The very best of humanity.

Then, the crowd parted.

Directly under the finish arch, holding my fiftieth state medal, was David. *My person.*

I could see the tears in his eyes as he bent down to place the medal around my neck.

He knelt down to look into my eyes. And the world stopped. Our lives are so short, yet this moment—thankfully and beautifully—stretched out right there for us, for a lifetime. A hush fell over the crowd. He cupped my face, exactly the way he had at our wedding, and kissed me. I grabbed him around the neck, laughing and crying in equal measure, as he buried his face in my hair.

We came apart, laughing and wiping tears from each other's eyes.

I told him I wouldn't cry. Oh, well. I was wrong—and refuse to feel guilty about it.

⁓

I stayed parked in front of the finish arch for a long time, getting hugged and smiling for photos.

Dad, tears in his eyes, said, "I am just so proud of you." His voice choked with emotion. He has always done his best to love and protect me. That's what parents should do. And I have grown to appreciate him for that. Oh, and after Alaska, Dad got his very first tattoo—a swallow, of course. At age eighty, he's finally a fucking rebel.

Then Mom. We hugged, hard. She had a hip replacement scheduled in her near future, but she also had a goal: to work her way back to a 5K after the surgery. She's tough and loving—a perfect paradox. I admire her more now than ever.

A young girl, about ten years old, came up to my trike and handed me a note. She had heard my talk at her school. Her note said I gave her hope for her big sister who had leukemia. A high school student who had also heard me speak at his school presented me with a homemade metal sign that read GO ON BE BRAVE—detailed with flying swallows. *The message had landed.*

In fact, the entire POW community seemed to embrace my message about bravery, community, and Hope. David described the trip as a "weeklong hug." A hug no one wanted to end, apparently, because we've both been invited back as the guest speakers for the 2023 marathon. (I think they just want to see the documentary!)

Finally, Dr. Bedlack walked up to me and stuck out his fist for a bump.

He said, "You just accomplished something I didn't think was possible."

In the beginning of the Team Drea Challenge in 2015, I had said: "There is nothing like crossing the finish line of a race you weren't sure you could finish." The moment that cracks open your self-imposed limitations on what is possible? Well, it changes everything.

At the finish line of Alaska, I understood why:

Nothing is impossible with Hope.

Hope, it turns out, is a pretty badass fighter.

CHAPTER 36

TWENTY-TWO
TRUTHS

1. Nietzsche and Kelly Clarkson were wrong. What doesn't kill you can only make you stronger if you learn the lesson from the experience. Otherwise, it'll just beat you down.

2. No matter what doctors or medical literature says, neither can predict your future.

3. Hopelessness will kill you faster than any disease will.

4. You can be depressed, or you can live your life. The time will pass either way.

5. You can exceed all self-imposed limitations.

6. Why take unnecessary risks? Because that's where the beauty of life is.

7. Life is so temporary. But it always continues.

8. We're all flying on one engine whether we know it or not.

9. "When we focus on *being* instead of *doing*, we don't need to define our value by how productive we are. *Who we are* shapes what we choose to do."—Beth, life coach extraordinaire

10. Everything does not happen for a reason. Things happen, and it's up to us to give that thing a reason. To lend our perspective. To make something meaningful out of tragedy. To help others in ways that we

can, and they cannot. This is how we express our appreciation for the gifts we have. This is what makes us *human*.

11.   "Whatever you do, get it on film."—Jon Blais
12.   "Until further notice, celebrate everything."—Arthur Cohen
13.   Tomorrow is not promised. It never was.
14.   What really matters is what we choose to do with the time that we have.
15.   You can say anything in your head, as long as what comes out is kind.
16.   "Your body is always trying to heal itself."—Mom
17.   Your mom was not/is not always wrong.
18.   Guilt is a wasted emotion.
19.   One foot in front of the other. When that's too much—stop, reset, and find the right impetus to keep fighting. Any forward progress is enough. One hard day, Hope will fight its way right into becoming *Belief*.
20.   Find joy in the struggle. Be scared and go for it anyway.
21.   Nothing is impossible with Hope. Hope is a pretty badass fighter.
22.   Go on, be brave. End ALS.

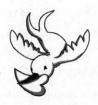

EPILOGUE

In July 2016 Andrea and I traveled to Hendersonville, North Carolina, to host an ALS fundraiser alongside the co-owners of Sanctuary Brewing Company, a local brewery. The brewery was nestled in the southern mountains of the western part of the state, and we had no connection to the area other than a friend, Andrew, who had been instrumental in setting up the fundraiser.

As Andrea and I spoke with the owners of Sanctuary and thanked them for hosting the event, my eyes were continually drawn to a group that had huddled several tables together. The younger man seated at the head of the tables held court among the boisterous group playing cornhole, giving belly rubs to dogs passing by, and laughing alongside him.

The young man's name was Tim. He sat in a motorized wheelchair that I recognized as similar to the model Andrea had gotten soon after we moved down to North Carolina. His wiry legs and arms showed the hallmark signs of atrophy. He would have towered over us if he had the strength to stand, I thought.

He smiled with a big, toothy grin. He appeared to be on the receiving end of loving barbs from the crowd of friends and family; I imagined they provided him with plenty of reasons to grin. When we met him, he and Andrea connected over their shared experience, making jokes that made us laugh, as well as fight back tears.

"Having my toes stretched"—he paused to ensure he maintained his captive audience—"is better than sex." His delivery of the line was brilliant and showed zero signs of atrophy.

As we made our way around his table, I met Tim's mother.

"You know, this is the first time he has left the house since he was diagnosed," she said.

"How long ago was he diagnosed?" I asked.

"About three years," she replied.

Three years, I thought. *Three years inside with ALS. This isn't just the body succumbing to the disease. His mind yielded before his muscles have, and there is no wheelchair for a broken spirit.*

"He had always been so social before his diagnosis. After he got sick, he didn't want to see anyone," another family member chimed in. His mother appeared to drift off while thinking about the last three years.

But in a beat, she returned to the conversation.

"He didn't want to see anyone—until today," she said, gazing at her son warmly.

❧

When I think about Andrea's message of giving ourselves space to be hopeful, I think of this trip to Hendersonville. It reminds me that bravery comes in all forms. It shows me that two people who initially have polar opposite responses to the same diagnosis can eventually find a shared sense of community and courage.

But most urgently, it reminds me how many others are likely out there, allowing perceived limitations in their lives—whether they be ALS-related limitations or otherwise—to build walls within their own minds and between themselves and those who love them. Their stories and Andrea's story are linked, whether they are aware of it or not.

This disease is unrelenting. Her speech slows just a bit more with each passing week, and fatigue sets in more quickly as she tries to keep up her ordinary routine. On a daily basis, she encounters the push-and-pull of keeping herself strong by enervating core muscle groups while feeling other muscles exhaust themselves more quickly. She continues to trike and race, although she sees the horizon of her athletic journey more clearly than before. As exciting as our journey of the past three years has been, there have certainly been times where I've felt like I'm in a scramble to outpace a cresting wave, clinging to the hope that we'll eventually be able to find safe harbor as I resist the urge to peek back at what might one day soon crash down upon us.

Of course, as I've come to realize, Andrea *is* that safe harbor for me. Just as we have leaned on each other to navigate the darkest parts of our lives, Andrea's words will always be here for me to revisit, no matter what lies ahead. She has done more than help preserve my own memory of the last decade—and she has preserved *her memory* of the journey, which is the greatest gift that she could ever give me.

You see, the world through her eyes is an absolutely marvelous place. I have always known this, and I have always loved this about her, although it has become more true, more vibrant, and more pronounced with every passing day.

Despite life's inescapable bad luck, sorrow, and tragedy, she transforms: a car ride into an adventure, a project into a cause, a routine into a gift, and a to-do list into a legacy. If I could wish one thing for you, it would be that you find someone who fundamentally changes the way you see the world in the way Andrea has for me.

David Peet
January 21, 2023

THE 50 (51) MARATHONS

#	State	Race	Date	City, State
1	North Carolina	City of Oaks	11/1/2015	Raleigh, NC
2	Virginia	Shamrock Marathon	3/20/2016	Virginia Beach, VA
3	Ohio	Columbus Marathon	10/21/2018	Columbus, OH
4	South Carolina	Charleston Marathon	1/12/2019	Charleston, SC
5	Texas	Austin Marathon	2/17/2019	Austin, TX
6	Georgia	Publix Atlanta Marathon	3/17/2019	Atlanta, GA
7	Tennessee	Rock 'n' Roll Nashville	4/27/2019	Nashville, TN
8	Kentucky	Horse Capital Marathon	5/18/2019	Lexington, KY
9	Connecticut	Mainly Marathons-CT	6/24/2019	Simsbury, CT

10	Colorado	Aspen Valley Marathon	7/13/2019	Aspen, CO
11	Hawaii	Maui Marathon	10/13/2019	Ka'anapali, HI
12	Pennsylvania	Philadelphia Marathon	11/24/2019	Philadelphia, PA
13	Alabama	Rocket City Marathon	12/14/2019	Huntsville, AL
14	Arizona	Buckeye Marathon	1/4/2020	Buckeye, AZ
15	Louisiana	Rock 'n' Roll New Orleans	2/9/2020	New Orleans, LA
16	Mississippi	Mississippi Blues Marathon	2/29/2020	Jackson, MS
17	Arkansas	Little Rock Marathon	3/1/2020	Little Rock, AR
18	Idaho	Bear Lake Trifecta-ID	8/13/2020	St. Charles, ID
19	Wyoming	Bear Lake Trifecta-WY	8/14/2020	Cokeville, WY
20	Utah	Bear Lake Trifecta-UT	8/15/2020	Garden City, UT
21	Indiana	Fair on the Square Marathon	9/12/2020	Danville, IN
22	Illinois	Dam Site Run	10/25/2020	Hudson, IL
23	Kansas	Little Apple Marathon	10/31/2020	Manhattan, KS
24	Missouri	Bass Pro Conservation Marathon	11/1/2020	Springfield, MO
25	Florida	Sandy Claus Run	12/6/2020	Ponte Vedra, FL
26	Maryland	Salisbury Marathon	4/3/2021	Salisbury, MD

27	Rhode Island	Rhode Races-Newport	4/17/2021	Newport, RI
28	Washington	Windermere Marathon	5/16/2021	Spokane, WA
29	Oregon	Willamette Valley Marathon	5/23/2021	Salem, OR
30	Montana	Frank Newman Marathon	5/29/2021	Bozeman, MT
DNF	~~Massachusetts~~	Mainly Marathons-MA	6/13/2021	Chicopee, MA
31	Vermont	Mainly Marathons-VT	6/14/2021	Springfield, VT
32	New Hampshire	Mainly Marathons-NH	6/15/2021	Claremont, NH
33	Maine	Mainly Marathons-ME	6/16/2021	Sanford, ME
34	Michigan	MISH Waterfront Marathon	6/26/2021	Gladstone, MI
35	Wisconsin	Mainly Marathons-WI	7/15/2021	Sparta, WI
36	Minnesota	Mainly Marathons-MN	7/16/2021	St. Cloud, MN
37	Iowa	Main to Main Marathon	8/21/2021	Osage, IA
38	West Virginia	Moonlight on the Falls Marathon	8/28/2021	Davis, WV
39	Nebraska	Mainly Marathons-NE	9/14/2021	Chadron, NE
40	South Dakota	Mainly Marathons-SD	9/16/2021	Belle Fourche, SD
41	North Dakota	Mainly Marathons-ND	9/17/2021	Bowman, ND

42	Massachusetts	Martha's Vineyard Marathon	9/25/2021	Martha's Vineyard, MA
43	Oklahoma	Oklahoma City Memorial Marathon	10/3/2021	Oklahoma City, OK
44	New Jersey	Atlantic City Marathon	10/17/2021	Atlantic City, NJ
45	New Mexico	Mainly Marathons-NM	11/7/2021	Farmington, NM
46	Delaware	Coastal Delaware Running Festival	11/12/2021	Rehoboth Beach, DE
47	Nevada	Lake Mead Marathon	1/8/2022	Lake Mead National Recreation Area, NV
48	California	Oakland Marathon	3/20/2022	Oakland, CA
(51)	Boston	"My Own Boston Marathon"	4/17/22	Boston, MA
49	New York	Brooklyn Marathon	4/24/2022	Brooklyn, NY
50	Alaska	POW Marathon	5/28/2022	Craig, AK

ACKNOWLEDGMENTS

From Andrea

If I started individually naming all the people who made this book possible, my acknowledgements would stretch on longer than the manuscript itself. I can never adequately repay all the kindness and generosity that has been bestowed on me—all I can do is try to pay it forward in all the ways that I can, for as long as I can. If we have shared a laugh, a race, a beer, or a tattoo, please know that I have treasured it—and *you*.

To Team Drea, the POW community, race directors who believe in inclusion, Prolyfyck, and the donors who have contributed to ALS research: thank you for inspiring me to keep going, and stepping up over and over again.

To MJ McSpadden and Brian Beckman: thank you for jumping into the documentary with no plan or budget, for being willing to make it up as we go, and for seeing it through. It is truly the most incredible gift. Sorry (not sorry) for all the running!

To my parents: thank you for always being proud of me, and being there every single time I needed you in the best way you knew how.

To Meredith: thank you for being relentlessly patient, relentlessly positive, and relentless with the edit pen.

To David: thank you for being my person. I love every single adventure with you.

To the women of Her ALS Story: thank you for being the group I had been searching for all along.

To the ALS community: if you are fighting this disease or loving someone who is, know that your story is not written—only you can do that. If you are a researcher or have lost your loved one to ALS, thank you for staying in the fight—we need you now more than ever.

From Meredith

Through this book (and the film), my family now knows the magic of Andrea Peet. Her contagious wisdom and joy. The gritty, scrappy, and powerful Hope she radiates. And I hope the entire world learns of it too.

Hope Fights Back was a quiet little project that started organically.

Andrea: I'm working on my book. Will you be my writing coach?

Me: Yes.

Andrea: Maybe you can look at what I've written?

Me: Yes.

Andrea: What did you think?

Me: Let's just do this thing together. The whole book.

Andrea: Yes, let's.

And really, that's how it went—paraphrased for emphasis and brevity. But it didn't take much arm twisting from either of us. Suddenly, I was *in* this book with Andrea.

Here's why. You do not stand in a doorway with Andrea Peet and say, "Eh, maybe I'll just stay here and help—a little . . ."

No, you go *through the door with her*. To wherever she points. Because that's *who* she is.

And what you *do* with that casual point or push from Andrea? Well, that is the answer of who *you* are.

For me, the book required that I find odd hours between the law job I had returned to, as well as intense focus. I struggled at the outset, because her purpose, words, and fight were now partially in my hands. *Hope Fights Back* deserved much more thought, reverence, and space than anything I had ever written about bikes, porta-potties, and *Nonsense*-eradicating behaviors.

It required a lot of tissues. Sometimes denial, too.

For months and months, I sat back, worked on the project, and set up a wall. I willed myself to *forget* that Andrea was, in fact, dying. Even in editing her very clear story.

But "life is not a dress rehearsal," so I slowly began to wake up.

The book addresses the brutality of ALS, but honestly, it does not scratch the surface of how devastating this disease really is. We omitted some of the brutality, because, well, we wanted you to also *like* the book—not put it in the freezer like Joey did on that *Friends* episode when he was scared of his Stephen King book.

And if you like this book, you'll tell your friends, you'll host book clubs, and someone who personally knows Oprah or Reese will make the call. . . And that's how *Hope Fights Back* will sell millions of copies and, in turn, raise millions of dollars for ALS research. *Goals.*

In December 2022, Stella (my daughter) and I spent a weekend in Raleigh with Andrea to work on the book.

Andrea and I worked so damn hard all weekend. I swear we sat at a table for three days and barely moved except for typing and talking. Stella and I shared meals with Andrea and David. We laughed (a lot), mostly at Stella hiding from the meal delivery folks every time they walked by, dropping smoothies and salads at the door. We brainstormed. We worked harder. *Apparently, my family way, too.*

And I, apparently, *hovered.*

I hovered around the delicacy of David and Andrea's well-perfected life dance—their love, their movements, their silent language. I hovered while Andrea maneuvered her walker, navigating the so-called accessible VRBO I had picked (*not quite, VRBO*).

But she navigated fine—of course, you've read this book—you know she did. Anytime David was at the house, he wasn't hovering. I tried to take a lesson from him, making mental notes of how to be, and how to be helpful.

But I still hovered.

After David and Andrea left for the night, Stella picked up the printed draft of the first few pages and read it. She made a face.

"Oh no! What?" I asked my thirteen-year-old, horrified.

Stella said, "No, it's good . . . but . . . you need a hook for this start! You need to pull the reader in fast—like Colleen Hoover does!" (Colleen Hoover is a fiction writer. But she was onto something.)

I looked at the first few pages.

Stella was right. I handed her the paper and said, "You are correct. Write it." Her eyes were big, but she gladly took the pen and pages. And at thirteen years old, she took off writing her revisions of the intro titled "ALS" . . . and she nailed the concept.

The next day, I showed Andrea.

Andrea's eyes sparkled, and she said, "I love it."

Which shows just who Andrea is—again—giving someone, even a youngster, the air under her little wings to pursue a dream. A few months later, James (our fifteen-year-old son) made some digital drawings of Andrea's swallow tattoos as an option for the interior book art. She said she loved them. So that is the bird art you see in this book. She just continues to be the *cheerleader for humanity*.

Before we headed back to Atlanta, Andrea told David, "I want Meredith to see our house so she has some perspective on our lives."

At the same moment she spoke these words, Andrea was literally *trapped* in her pullover jacket that David was helping her put on. Her head and arms were stuck.

David said, "I don't think she needs more perspective than this."

At which point—still trapped in her jacket—Andrea's laugh filled the room, and we all followed suit.

Stella and I walked Andrea to her car on the last day. No David that day, just the girls. She hugged me big before getting into her car. She promptly folded and put her walker in the passenger seat.

I stood there.

She then said, "You are hovering."

We laughed again. (And I may have hovered another few bonus seconds.)

I *was* hovering. And she didn't need me to do anything except get out of her way . . . and drive back to Atlanta to work on the edits of our incredibly aggressive, record-setting-in-the-world-of-publishing manuscript turnaround time. (Seriously, if I told you how hard and fast this all happened—no publishing house would actually believe it. Thank you, Pegasus and Jessica!)

Paradoxically, I had been depressed most of 2022. Sort of ridiculous to find yourself depressed working on a project like this. But I was. I acknowledge it. *Guilt is a waste of time.*

So, in this acknowledgment, I further acknowledge *Hope*, in all its glory. I have received a strong wave of my own Hope returning and fighting back. I am more myself today than I've been before Andrea's words. Because that's what Andrea encourages.

With this book project, I learned to engage in life again, to straighten some of my Nonsense out, and to move forward. And that's because of you, Andrea. You *are* Hope.

And oh, how much I love you, Andrea Lytle Peet! Thank you for letting me co-pilot this book—a book that was always flying on two perfect engines, with or without my help. Of course, thank you, David, for your amazing role in this project and for allowing the Locks to let the light in.

To Jason, James IV, and Stella Rae—I love you so much. Jason—your one file folder allows me to do what matters, and I am so appreciative. James—your swallow art is perfect for this book! Your talents are such a gift—thank you for sharing them. So proud of you. Stella—your contribution to the voice of this book and your pre-reading is priceless. Although Door Dash called, and they're still looking for you.

Thank you to Brent Pease and Kyle Pease (the Kyle Pease Foundation) for being exactly who you are; Jay Holder of the Atlanta Track Club; CrossFit Dwala for being my satellite office; Judy Newberry for your support and understanding as I navigate between life, law, and writing; and Todd Nixon for yet another book pre-read and all your chips; and always, BEE: Renee Sedliar—my forever all-things-books-and-words friend. To the rest of my family—love to you all—thanks for being enthusiastic about everything, always.

A thank you from Andrea and me both to: Pegasus Books for believing in Andrea's story and agreeing to the speedy turnaround time to make it happen, Eryn Kalavsky (our agent), Jessica Case (our editor), Meghan Jusczak (our publicist), and Beth Helfrich (our extra set of editing eyes).

Now, off to Be Brave, End ALS . . . and buy that damn boat.

Please consider buying your TEN favorite friends a copy of this book, purchasing copies for your local library or favorite organization, sharing on social media, and also making a donation in Andrea's honor: www.TeamDrea.org.

NOTES

ALS

1. "Amyotrophic Lateral Sclerosis: Diagnosis," Muscular Dystrophy Association, https://www.mda.org/disease/amyotrophic-lateral-sclerosis/diagnosis.

CHAPTER 2

1. https://www.dictionary.com/e/slang/what-doesnt-kill-you-makes-you-stronger/.

CHAPTER 9

1. "Working Together to Educate People about ALS," ALS Association, May 4, 2021, https://www.als.org/blog/working-together-educate-people-about-als.
2. "How Long Can You Live with ALS? Amyotrophic Lateral Sclerosis (ALS) Life Expectancy," Very Well Health, February 17, 2023, https://www.very wellhealth.com/als-lou-gehrigs-disease-life-expectancy-2223973.
3. More recent studies have concluded that exercise is moderately beneficial to people with ALS. Frank Greenwood, "Exercise and ALS: Some of the Latest Research," ALS Therapy Development Institute, September 21, 2020, https://www.als.net/news/excercise-and-als-some-of-the-latest-research.

CHAPTER 11

1. Anthony Carbajal, "ALS Ice Bucket Challenge—Uncensored & Sexy?" YouTube, August 18, 2014, https://www.youtube.com/watch?v=h07OT8p8Oik.
2. "Full Text of Lou Gehrig's Farewell Speech," *Sports Illustrated*, July 4, 2009, https://www.si.com/mlb/2009/07/05/gehrig-text.

CHAPTER 18

1. S. Padilla, "A Quick History of Wheelchair Racing," WheelchairParts.net, June 12, 2020, https://wheelchairparts.net/blog/a-quick-history-on-wheelchair-racing.
2. Michael Weinreib, "Wheelchair Racers Split, with Organizers in Middle," *New York Times*, November 2, 2006, https://www.nytimes.com/2006/11/02/sports/sportsspecial/02handcycle.html.

3. Jon Marcus, "Missoula Marathon Settles Discrimination Case," *Runner's World*, February 5, 2016, https://www.runnersworld.com/news/a20860677/missoula-marathon-settles-discrimination-case.

4. *News & Observer*, October 19, 2017, https://www.newsobserver.com/latest-news/article179681776.html.

5. Steve Hartman, "N.C. Man Bakes Up Krispy Kreme Caper," CBS News, January 3, 2014, https://www.cbsnews.com/news/nc-man-bakes-up-krispy-kreme-caper.

CHAPTER 25

1. The Kyle Pease Foundation has the mission to "Improve the lives of people with disabilities through sports" and "create opportunities of inclusion for every person with a disability." "The Foundation," https://www.kylepeasefoundation.org/aboutkpf.

CHAPTER 27

1. "A truly inclusive marathon provides space for every runner to register, compete and be celebrated exactly as they are," said Joanna Hoffman, spokesperson for Athlete Ally, a group that advocates for LGBTQI+ equality in sports. Joe Hernandez, "Runners Can Identify as Non-binary in the Boston and London Marathons," NPR, April 17, 2023, https://www.npr.org/2022/09/14/1123035038/nonbinary-runners-boston-london-marathon.

2. "Official Charity Program of the Boston Marathon," BAA, https://www.baa.org/races/boston-marathon/charity-program.

3. Tish Hamilton, "Life of a BQ Squeaker," *Runner's World*, June 25, 2018, https://www.runnersworld.com/runners-stories/a21288665/life-bq-squeaker.

4. Charlie Watson, "How People Are Running the Boston Marathon without a BQ," *Women's Running*, February 8, 2017, https://www.womensrunning.com/training/road/run-boson-marathon-without-bq.

CHAPTER 33

1. Boston's new categories aligned with the ten classifications of the Paralympic Games. "IPC Classification," IPC International Paralympic Committee, https://www.paralympic.org/classification.

2. As Marla Runyan, then para athlete manager for the BAA and a blind runner herself, explained about the new Adaptive Program: "You have an elite field, you have an emerging elite field, you have athletes aspiring to run their personal best, and you have charity runners running for a cause—you have the full range of folks racing with different motivations and different athletic abilities, and that same continuum exists among the para athlete community." Allison Torres Burtka, "Recognizing Competition, Boston Adds Para Athletics Divisions," Global Sports Matters, July 1, 2019, https://globalsportmatters.com/health/2019/07/01/recognizing-competition-boston-adds-para-athletic-divisions.

ABOUT THE AUTHORS

ANDREA LYTLE PEET (@teamdreafoundation) is an urban planner and triathlete who was diagnosed with ALS at the age of thirty-three. She began to write her story with the disease as it unfolded—in real time. Andrea and her husband, David, established the Team Drea Foundation which raises funds for ALS research. She is a graduate of Davidson College and Georgia Tech and currently lives in Raleigh, North Carolina with her husband and two cats.

MEREDITH ATWOOD (@Meredith.Atwood) is an attorney, author of *Triathlon for the Every Woman* and *The Year of No Nonsense*, four-time IRONMAN triathlete, and former host of *The Same 24 Hours* podcast. She is a graduate of the University of Georgia and lives in Roswell, Georgia with her husband, two teenagers, and one cat.